head massage

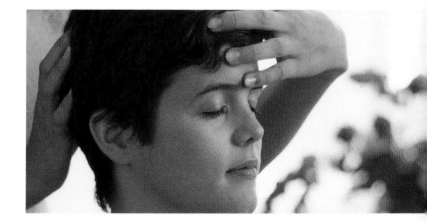

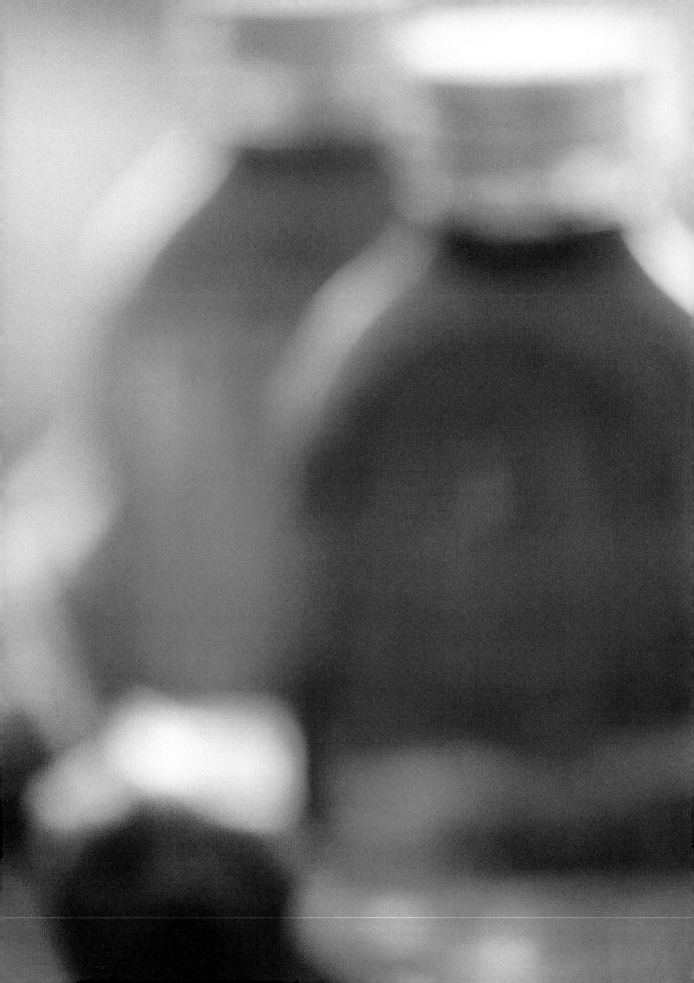

head massage

Rosalind Widdowson

hamlyn

Executive editor - **Jane McIntosh**
Assistant editor - **Sharon Ashman**
Creative art director - **Keith Martin**
Senior designer - **Claire Harvey**
Book design - **Martin Topping**
Production - **Lucy Woodhead**
Photography - **Jacqui Wornell**

First published in Great Britain in 2000 by Hamlyn, a division of Octopus Publishing Group Limited, 2–4 Heron Quays, London E14 4JP

Copyright © Octopus Publishing Group Limited 2000
ISBN 0 600 60054 8

A catalogue record for this book is available from the British Library

Produced by Toppan Printing Company Ltd
Printed in China

Distributed in the United States by Sterling Publishing Co., Inc. 387 Park Avenue South, New York, NY 10016-8810

contents

introduction

My early life was a rich tapestry of exploration and first-hand experiences. One of my first and most lasting memories was watching African babies being bathed in the river and then massaged with Vaseline until their skin shone in the sunlight. It had a profound effect upon me and I became fascinated by the way these mothers cared for and nurtured their offspring. Many of the women had to stand working for hours, either ironing, cooking or gardening. Their babies were gently bound around their middles with woollen blankets while they continued with their daily chores. In all my years of growing up in this environment I cannot remember any of the babies crying in distress. I feel sure it was their daily bath and massage ritual as well as the continued warmth and comfort of their mother's touch and repetitive movements which kept them all so happy and contented.

Touch has played a key role in all my work as a natural health consultant. I have developed self-help massage techniques to improve the quality of yoga practice as well as my Hi-Ki method of massage. The idea of head wrapping for clients who had difficulty in accepting touch, especially those who had been traumatized or who were in some kind of physical or emotional pain, has proved invaluable. This special technique is constantly evolving. I recently used it while working in a cancer clinic in Germany and have now incorporated it into my detox programmes along with my de-stress treatments.

My Hi-Ki approach was first inspired many years ago by Mahatma Gandhi's words: 'No culture can survive if it attempts to be exclusive.' This stimulated my interest in developing and integrating the many wonderful practices available throughout the world. In my travels I have been able to learn from many masters and expand the range of my techniques.

Fundamentally the principle of Hi-Ki is based on the balancing, not just of the body energies, but of the environment around the practice which both complements and reinforces the efficacy of the methods. By a form of osmosis we absorb the energies that surround us. Ultimately our work, rest and play are affected by the environment we inhabit.

The difference between that which is truly alive and that which is not is the presence or absence of that mystical force called *ki*, *chi* or *prana*. It is the energetic substratum and organizing intelligence. While we are alive *ki* permeates every part of our body, helping to maintain good bodily functions. The important function of the Hi-Ki form of massage is to stimulate the flow and proper direction of this life force throughout the body. The more *ki* that reaches the cells, the less prone to decay they will be. Unhealthy creatures are not vibrant because their *ki* is not flowing smoothly.

The main function of Hi-Ki is to help rebalance the flow, no matter what the outer circumstances or influences may be. The practitioner prepares the body and mind as well as the environment before the practice, and also performs a simple ritual of personal and environmental cleansing when the treatments are complete. These procedures are easy to follow as I have choreographed the basic techniques into routines that form a moving meditation. The more you practise, the more fine-tuned your touch will become. It will be like tuning a musical instrument, the melodies of which go far beyond the normal sounds and act on a subliminal level to heal both practitioner and recipient, and also create mental and physical space. Lines of worry can indeed be smoothed away by the power of touch and it is possible to sculpt a face of ageless beauty.

I have structured the book in such a way as to give you a grounding in techniques that are universally practised throughout a range of different cultures. Some still maintain and cultivate a self-empowering, low-technology form of home healthcare based around the family and community. The latter part of the book, however, introduces more advanced and subtle variations which acknowledge the reality of meridians and *chakra* energies.

Head massage is a perfect tool for easing mental stress which would otherwise be instrumental in causing serious long-term illnesses – depression and anxiety are the long-term killers. Within each and every one of us lies the power to heal. Our hands are the perfect instruments for that loving task and, with them, it is possible to help yourself and your loved ones to a better quality of health.

I have written this book after more than 35 years of inspired practice, using both the Oriental and Western classical practices. As the twenty-first century dawns I am looking forward to my forthcoming television series on natural health and inaugurating the first Hi-Ki teacher training courses. No doubt each day will continue to be a revelation and my teaching will also continue to change, incorporating features of which I am as yet unaware.

Head massage is a classic therapy yet it is kept ever-fresh by every student and practitioner who undertakes this noble art. Modern medicine is only now coming to realize the benefits of such complementary therapies in the overall wellbeing of its patients. We all look forward to the breaking down of previously restricted views and prejudices on the subject. As many people now realize, good health is not to be found solely in the pill-dispensing preserve of the allopathic medical professional. It is the responsibility of every one of us and I urge you to claim it.

I wish you all the very best in your pathway to health and happiness.

the origins and history of head massage

Massage can be traced back thousands of years and is probably one of the oldest therapies known to mankind. The earliest written testimony probably dates from 3000 BC. The Ayur Veda – the Indian scriptural text and foundation of Ayurvedic Medicine – was compiled around 1800 BC, and massage depictions appear on a number of ancient Egyptian temples and tombs.

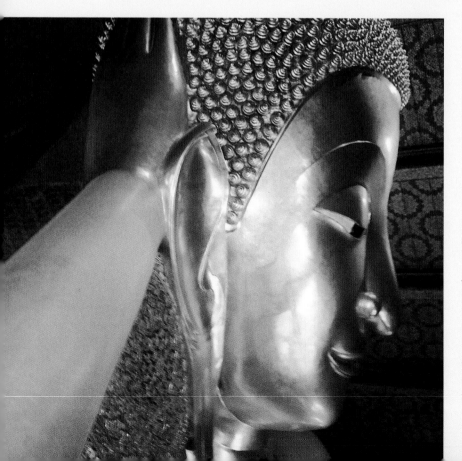

The Chinese *Nei Ching*, written 3000 years ago by the legendary 'Yellow Emperor', records in meticulous detail the classical theory and practice of Oriental medicine and includes many references to the art of massage. To the ancient Greek and Roman physicians, massage was one of the principal means of healing and relieving pain. In 500 BC, Hippocrates – the father of modern medicine – wrote: 'The physician must be experienced in many things, but assuredly in rubbing . . . For rubbing can bind a joint that is too loose, and loosen a joint that is too rigid'. Influential writers such as Socrates, Plato and Pliny the naturalist all wrote about and received massage treatments.

Massage and, in particular, the laying on of hands, is largely sanctioned by most religions and certainly features favourably in their texts. In the East it has always been considered an essential skill for medical practitioners and healers. Unfortunately the Middle Ages saw the custom fall into disuse due to the Christian contempt for the body and 'worldly pleasures'. Massage suffered as a result, only to reappear after the Renaissance. Only then were the ancient and still vital skills appreciated and acquired again by the West. Europe in general did not become reacquainted with the noble art until the Swede Per Henrik Ling introduced the systematic technique known as 'Swedish Massage'.

China, Japan, India, Egypt, Greece and Rome have all contributed their know-how and integrated systems to the fund of knowledge that forms the wellspring of the range of treatments that are on offer today. The moving meditation, with one movement blending into another, was developed as an art form with the introduction of plaiting and beading.

The remedial benefits of these fascinating practices form a fast-growing area in the world of self-help therapy. Head massage is the crowning glory of massage techniques. It offers the perfect tool for easing the mental stress which is instrumental in causing many serious long-term illnesses.

The core of head massage lies in its unique way of communicating without words. It is like entering a special room until now locked and hidden away, an inner sanctuary for the purpose of healing and recreation. On its own this state of rest is a wonderful experience, but consecutive treatments will do more, helping you to replenish and revive, melting away your stresses and strains.

Massage has a long history of tried and tested techniques developed throughout the world over thousands of years. The ancients knew how to use their hands as a tool to heal and treat long before allopathic medicine was even invented. Nowhere encapsulates the ancient tradition of head massage better than the Traditional Massage School at Wat Po in Bangkok, site of the famous Reclining Buddha. In its grounds are to be found the ancient texts and meridian diagrams so essential to the healer-practitioners and their tutors. Statues of the original Medicine Buddha adorn the grounds, their imagery instructive to both student and tourist alike. The school in Wat Po is a prime example of the ancient art of massage thriving in modern culture.

Below left: The Reclining Buddha, Wat Po, Bangkok, Thailand.

Below: Meridian diagrams on the walls of Wat Po's Traditional Massage School.

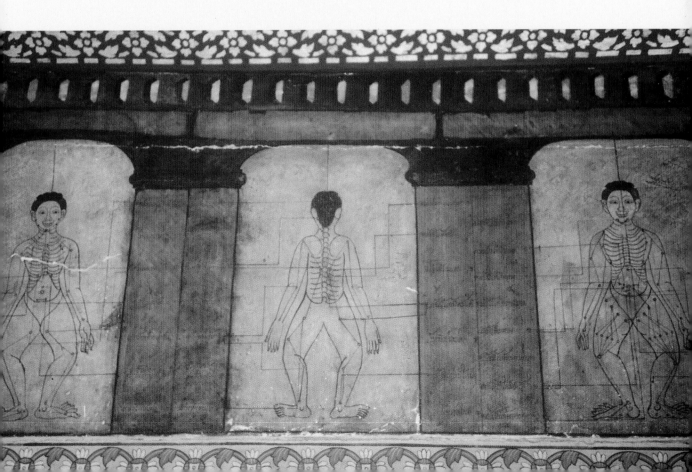

physical and mental benefits

The balancing art of massage offers a pathway to health and healing, and will enable you to begin living in harmony with Nature and your own unique constitution. The comprehensive listings below will give you some idea of its all-round effectiveness.

Addictions

Massage treatments work on the principle of reconnecting the recipient to the natural rhythms of life, restoring a sense of inner peace which awakens the flow of healing.

Ageing

Head massage arrests the ageing process by helping to keep the body and mind in tip-top working order.

AIDS

The special wrapping techniques which can benefit AIDS sufferers were pioneered in clinics in Thailand, St Lucia, Greece, Germany and England and can have great effect. In addition, the soothing, wave-like sounds of the massage strokes can evoke a feeling of comfort and calmness.

Bodily functions

Informed manipulation of specific pressure points can clear vital connections and ensure correct functioning, preventing and relieving everyday problems such as asthma, bronchitis, constipation, indigestion, blood pressure, skin disorders, and mental and physical distress.

Brain power

By unblocking the subtle lines of energy, head massage increases the supply of oxygen to the brain. Its tension-releasing abilities ensure that cortisone build-up does not shrink brain matter.

Cancer

Self-help healing and head wrapping can be a great comfort to those suffering from forms of this major illness.

Circulation

This is greatly improved, as are cold feet and hands, and chilblains. Head massage can also help to prevent cramps, PMT, menopausal symptoms, headaches and panic attacks.

Dandruff

Certain oils and regular practice will eliminate this minor problem.

Depression and anxiety

The whole body is like a complex computer: it memorizes all our pain and suffering. Within minutes, a practitioner can tune into bodily traumas and calm, soothe and draw away layers of discomfort. Touching through massage is a language all of its own. Touch is one of the first senses we develop and last senses to go, and can show love and healing in even traumatic circumstances.

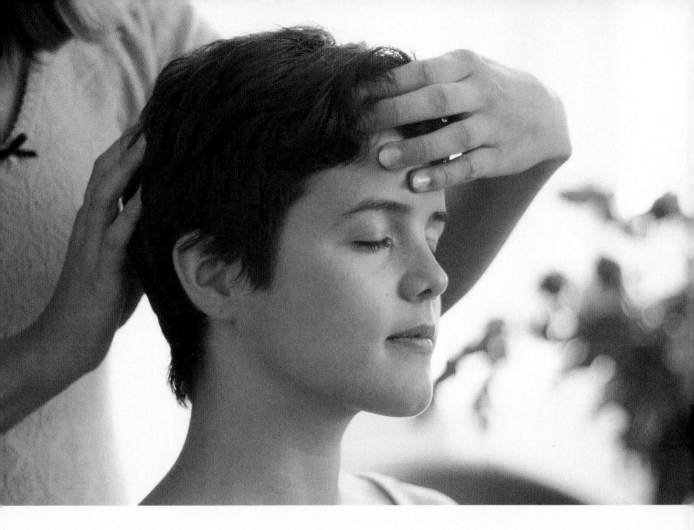

Diuretic process

Head massage stimulates the diuretic process – the discharge of urine – one of Nature's finest cleansers and detoxifying techniques. It activates the lymphatic system and helps clear blockages.

Electromagnetic energy

This is corrected by fine-tuned massage techniques.

Emotional trauma

This can be instantly arrested with sensitivity and care.

Hair and scalp

Head massage retards hair loss, premature balding and greying. It also corrects the balance of secretions and rebalances dry or oily scalps.

Headaches and migraines

Head massage can readjust the balance of pressures in the head, clearing sinuses, rebalancing synovial fluid, de-stressing neck and shoulder muscles, and relieving eyestrain.

Hormones

Certain practices that work on the third eye, the massage site of the pituitary gland – master regulator of our endocrine system – ensure the optimum working of this so-important gland.

Immune system

Clearing blockages increases the body's resistance to disease.

Mental clarity and focus

Soothing the senses helps to dispel unwanted thoughts, leaving the mind calm and clear.

Mind and memory

Stagnant *ki* is eliminated with special care and attention. The tendency to daydream is arrested by balanced massage movements and bodily alignment. These movements are like a moving meditation, a fine art which acts as a pathway to self-discovery and spiritual practice.

Natural face-lift

Your smile is the finest face-lift. Head massage will return that smile to replace anxious, tense, strained and tired expressions.

Nervous system

The elimination of fatigue and deep-seated stress and strain helps to soothe, relax and invigorate this complex working mechanism.

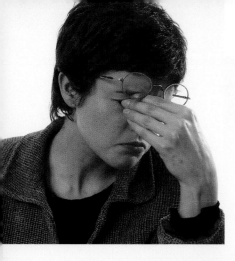

stressful living

Human beings were not designed for life in the twenty-first century. We have not evolved anything like quickly enough to deal with the demands of a fast-paced, information-rich, stressful environment. In evolutionary terms we are still in the Stone Age, perfectly adapted for the life of a hunter-gatherer, not that of a business executive or working mother.

Our endocrine system rules our lives very effectively by releasing hormones, chemical messengers that regulate our metabolism, moods, sexuality and survival responses. When the system is in proper balance we are positively oriented people with a curiosity and zest for life. When for any reason – physical, emotional or mental – that balance is disturbed and the functioning of the system becomes irregular, overproductive, damaged or has to run on overdrive for too long, then we are living stressed lives.

Modern life exposes us to a myriad of pressures, presenting problems which are often beyond our control. This produces a stress response from our endocrine system – a cocktail of hormones which prepare the body for physical or mental exertion. Unlike the short-term need of our ancestors, we are required to keep our systems in overdrive just to cope sometimes. The long-term effect is a condition called chronic stress. Continued high levels of the stress hormone cortisol suppress the immune response, making us particularly vulnerable to viral infections, and can lead to heart attacks, cancer and memory loss.

We can find ourselves living a stressful lifestyle without really being aware of it. The habit of living on a treadmill just to survive has become second nature to many of us. All thoughts of how we are really spending our time have been put to the backs of our minds.

Stress in the twenty-first century is going to be one of the primary causes of health breakdown. Stepping onto the treadmill of life is all too commonplace; slowing down and switching off is another matter. But there is no getting away from it: we all have to make choices on how to deal with the problem because our coping skills will ultimately fail us.

All too often, as the pace hots up, we respond to it with a reflex action of tightening our minds and bodies just to 'hold on' in order to protect our diminishing energy resources. The outward signs soon become plainly obvious . . . for example, more make-up masks, heavy metal jewellery, dark, heavier clothing, faster cars to get us to work 'on time'. We are so often oblivious to the image we have created in order to keep control.

Unfortunately the old adage of 'the more successful you become, the less healthy you are' turns out to be true and the idea that 'he who travels lightest travels furthest' becomes a pipedream. Our bodies become heavier with responsibility and our ever-increasing thought patterns. We are no longer able to walk lightly on the earth but instead grind our feet in to make our mark.

Living in the fast lane often means fast food – quick fixes of carbohydrates, fats, salt and sugar. We begin to drive ourselves to drink, then have to drug ourselves to get back on the road. The inevitable effects of stressful living will ultimately show in our faces, and in our hair which will no longer be our crowning glory. Put your hands into action with head massage and let them start to heal your life.

stressless living

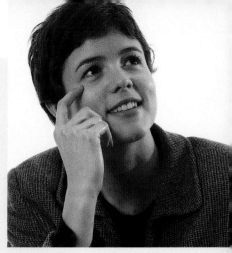

There are many helpful, well-recognized and approved methods of de-stressing and coming off the cycle of chronic stress. Below I outline just a few which I have found useful in my own life.

natural mental tonics

Worry and anxiety are a curse, especially to a person with lowered vitality and a gloomy outlook. From this moment onwards, determine that you are going to kick the worry habit. It only weakens the willpower, saps the nerves, unsteadies the thought patterns and ages the body. Worry is only a phantom of your imagination, it is not 'real' at all. Faith in yourself is sudden death to the worry demon. Consider the benefits of using positive affirmations such as: 'I will win through this crisis'; 'I am going to get well'; 'I am well'. Picture yourself as being perfectly fit and healthy: fit for anything, without a worry or a care in the world. Repeat these words to yourself every day in case you let things slide. This practice alone can work wonders and lead to stressless living.

Lighten up and laugh. When life threatens to overwhelm you there are two ways to deal with that energy. Habit patterns drive some people into depression and introspection. I prefer to see the funny side of things and to put a situation into the context of 'the bigger picture'. This produces an energy which is expansive, jovial and positively orientated, and its release often generates the overview that provides the very solution I need to find my way forward.

Relaxation and meditation are thoroughly proven methods of switching off from chronic stress and allowing our systems to calm down and recouperate.

Consider taking up a yoga class at least once a week. Alternatively, take advantage of some of the wonderful relaxation tapes and CDs on the market. Regular use of these techniques will create helpful patterns of behaviour and you will find that fewer things will irritate you or cause the stressed condition in the first place.

Co-listening (shared listening) is a well-recognized psychological tool. Having an outlet to express your thoughts, feelings, frustrations, and knowing that you are being heard is a most wonderful tonic. No one really teaches us how to listen and, because of that, we are always at risk of a breakdown in communication with our partners, siblings, friends, parents and colleagues. So often our inner voice is trying to speak to us and we ignore it, only to regret it later. Co-listening, in its many forms, is a valued source of learning how to listen, not just to other people but to ourselves.

natural physical tonics

A balanced programme of aerobic exercise and its complement, yoga or stretch-and-relax, are essential to a well-balanced lifestyle.

Regular or even occasional detoxification of the digestive and alimentary system is another traditionally recognized way of de-stressing an overworked and overloaded body. Therapies such as colonics and enemas can make the world of difference to one's energy levels and ability to deal with stress, and can prevent debilitating illness.

Eat more seasonal, local produce, preferably organic.

Start your day with a cup of hot, boiled water. Make sure your intake of fluid is sufficient and does not consist solely of toxin-laden, caffeine-rich drinks such as tea and coffee.

Ensure you find the time to take a breather. Literally take several deep breaths which fill the lower part of your lungs and expel stale air. Chair-bound office workers are so often in danger of decreased oxygen levels due to restricted seated positions and lack of exercise.

Wash away your worries at the beginning and end of the day. Couple your imagination and powers of visualization with the physical act of washing itself (see the waterfall, page 31). Clear away the clutter. Feng Shui – space clearing – is the best way to create sacred spaces in your work and home environment.

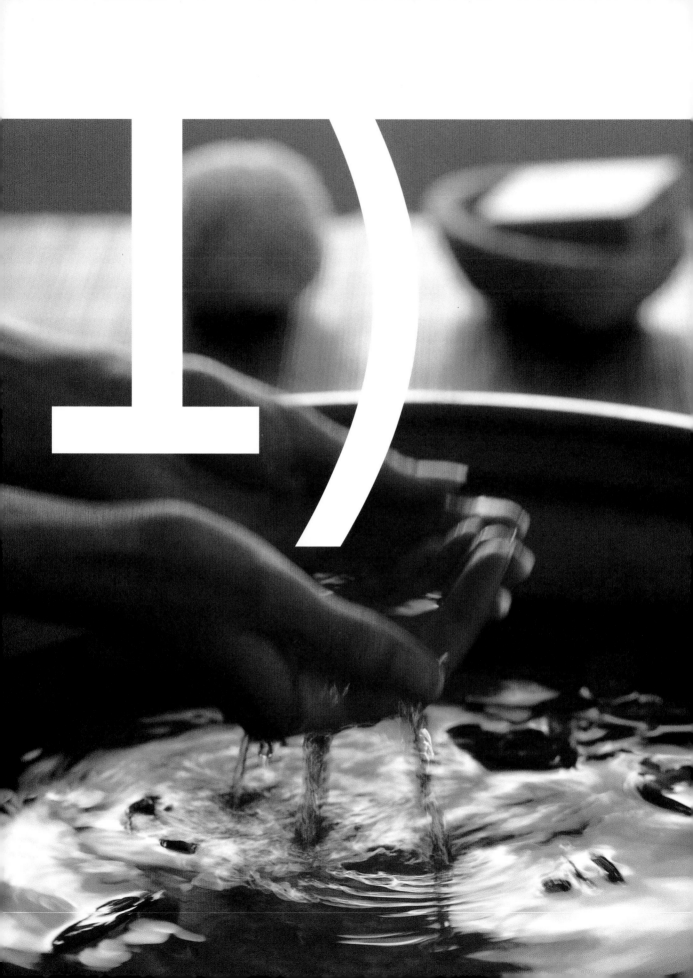

hi-ki getting started

creating a healing environment

A number of key elements will ensure a trouble-free session of head massage and provide a pleasant and memorable experience for your partner. The importance of creating a sympathetic healing environment can not be stressed enough – ringing phones, draughts, interruptions, unsympathetic lighting and so on can ruin an otherwise immensely enjoyable experience.

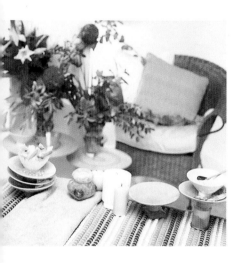

Above: Natural fabrics in subtle and muted tones, flowers and plants aid reconnection with the healing spirit.

Opposite: In order to achieve the best results your partner should be comfortably seated or lying in a well-balanced pose in a sympathetic environment.

Choice of working options

The main options for a surface on which to massage are discussed overleaf. However, make your choice after careful experimentation. The important thing is that you have ready access to your partner without the risk of back or knee strain; your partner should be comfortably seated or lying in a well-balanced pose. Do not be persuaded to offer treatment outside your own sympathetic environment if you know the set-up to be truly unfavourable.

A quiet and peaceful environment

Ensure that you choose a time and place which is unlikely to suffer interruptions or distractions during the session. Switch off all unnecessary electrical equipment, put the telephone on mute and divert calls to your answerphone or call service. Above all, prise your partner free of their mobile phone and place it out of reach and earshot. Allow at least 45 minutes for a full treatment.

Music

It seems silence is a rare commodity nowadays. Our private and public places are bombarded by an aural barrage.

Head massage is a very sensitive form of treatment and the natural sounds made by the working hands can themselves be considered part of the therapy. Whether or not to have music is your partner's choice, but if they do want it I suggest one of the inspirational CDs of natural sounds or sympathetically crafted mood albums as accompaniment. If you become familiar with an album it can offer you clues to the passage of time and the progress of your treatment.

Temperature and ventilation

Your working environment needs to be about 21°C (70°F) or warmer if you are working on the floor. Ventilation is necessary, particularly if you are burning incense, but make sure that there are no draughts. Whenever possible, work in the fresh air.

Lighting

Natural filtered light is by far the best medium. As an alternative, candles create a wonderfully evocative mood, even in daylight. At night, low, indirect lighting or candles are essential to create a suitable atmosphere. Avoid over-bright, glaring or insensitive lighting.

Room cleansing

As outlined on page 30, 'smudging' is a traditional method of both physically and psychically cleansing an environment. With any burning medium, be it smudging or incense burning, allow time for the smoke to clear or settle before you begin your treatment.

Removing clutter

Remove from the room any superfluous items, particularly ones that remind your partner of work or the environment they have just come from. This may include shoes, coats, briefcases and handbags. Work in as clear a space as possible, free from unnecessary clutter.

Bed linen

My recommendation is to use only natural fabrics for your sheets, pillows, blankets and wrapping cloths. Non-allergenic covers are also available. Whenever possible, use items which generate a sense of luxury. Warm the covers if it is cold and even provide a hot water bottle to cuddle for comfort, if necessary.

Essential oils and lotions

Head massage does not necessarily require oils and lotions. However, the back, neck and shoulders always feel better when worked with aromatherapy lotions. These are usually premixed with low levels of active essential ingredients and are largely safe for most people. They are readily available and easier to use than essential or carrier oils when you are first learning. Remember to pre-warm their containers and contents prior to treatment. Keep a selection of different lotions to hand and offer your partner their choice of fragrance.

Creating a sacred focal point

Set aside an area for a notable centrepiece as a focal point. Incorporate a range of natural elements such as flowers, plants and natural artefacts reflecting the five elements of Chinese tradition: metal, wood, water, fire and earth. The effect of such a simple finishing touch is often out of all proportion to the effort expended in creating it, for it encourages your partner to view your massage session as special and out of the ordinary, thus enhancing its therapeutic value.

Outdoor settings

Massaging in an outdoor setting can, on occasion, be problematical but the rewards are well worth it. The evocative pleasure of a shady tree or riverside sounds doubly enhances the head massage experience.

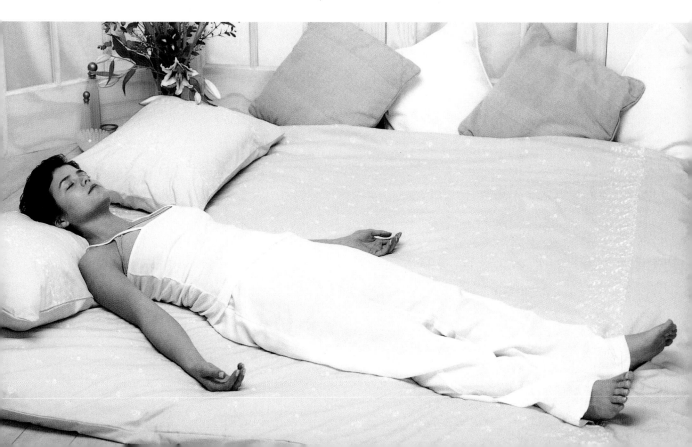

working options

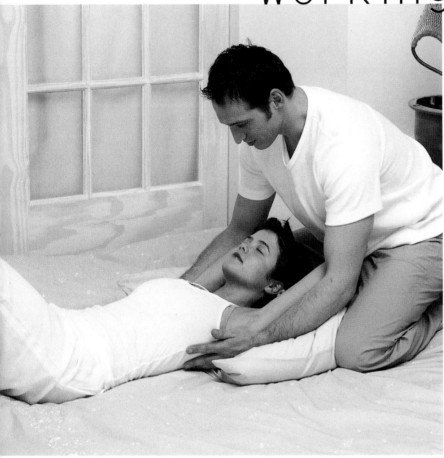

Above: A bed made up on the floor is a perfectly acceptable working option.

Standard bed

You can adapt and use any standard bed which is not encumbered with a head- or baseboard. Failing that, consider orientating your partner crossways on a double bed. Since this is not the ideal height, you will probably need to use a stool or to kneel on a firm cushion when working this way. You are unlikely to be able to get your knees under the bed allowing you to get close enough to your partner, so your practice might seem rather awkward. However, a standard bed is quite an acceptable option for short remedial treatments when other alternatives are simply not available, or your partner is already in bed. It also has the advantage of requiring little preparation and no clearing away after. In addition, most bedrooms are designed with relaxation in mind and have indirect lighting, which should only reinforce the effectiveness of your treatment.

Massage couch

There is no getting away from the fact that the massage couch is the ideal height and construction – that's why professionals use them. Higher than the standard bed, it allows you to get your legs and knees under the couch and intimately close to your partner when techniques demand. It also makes it easy to work on all four sides and at any height from sitting to standing. Whether purchased or homemade, the couch must be sturdy and impart confidence to whoever is trusting their

Floor

Making up a bed on the floor, if you have the space, gives ready access to the whole body. It allows your partner to let go fully, giving in to the pull of gravity, and thus achieve complete relaxation. There is also a sense of security in feeling connected to the earth, with no fear of falling due to inattention or drowsiness – something that can be a factor for those nervous of letting go.

The potential disadvantage to the masseur of this working option is that it limits certain types of movement or techniques which would need to be adapted for the prone position. In addition the masseur needs quite a flexible back to deal with the extra bending and manipulation required. However, any initial awkwardness should readily yield to practice and familiarization with the routines.

weight and security to it. I have known people use wallpaper-pasting tables with disastrous consequences. Personally I find most couches a little too narrow, but then there is usually a slight trade-off between access for you, the masseur, and ideal comfort for your partner.

Stool

A stool, or pair of adjustable stools, offers an excellent alternative to the prone position. Benefits include a chance to assess and correct postural alignment – so often the cause of head, neck and shoulder tension – and to gain good, all-round access and height differential. Indian head massage techniques favour the masseur's position at least a head or two higher than that of their partner. This is particularly important when you are using your body as both a back and head support, and performing cradling and cherishing movements. There is a lot of comfort to be derived by both masseur and recipient in this most nourishing and

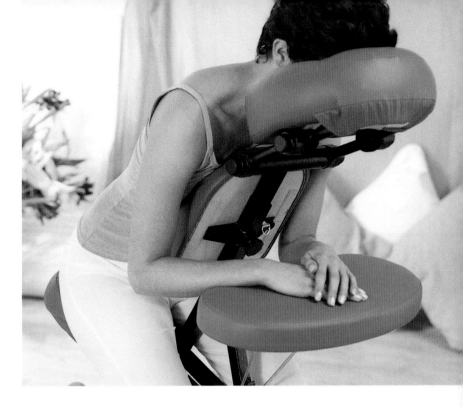

Above: The on-site massage chair is simply the ideal choice for both the professional or practitioner who wants to share their skills on a regular basis.

intimate arrangement. Since, in the absence of a chair back, you are the sole support, it is vital that you provide some kind of hand contact at all times. If you want to encourage your partner to relax and close their eyes, you must be their 'orienteer' and give them confidence during the massage.

Table and chair

For 'instant' treatments which can be accomplished in the typical home or office environment, you can do little better than a standard table and chairs. Most tables are manufactured or crafted at a standard height of 75 cm (30 in) and most accompanying chair sets have reasonable backrests. With the simple addition of a large pillow or cushion to support the chest and a rolled towel to support the head, you have a perfectly adequate massage position. There are, however, limitations and restrictions. Your partner's abdomen will be rather restricted and under pressure, so vary your movements and sequences to allow a period of upright release. Considering the width of most

tables and desks, you will be unable to perform certain techniques that require you to work in front of your partner, although some adaptations can be made.

On-site massage chair

Finally, the ideal – the professional, purpose-built, on-site portable massage chair. It gives all-round access, and your partner is in a perfectly balanced and unrestricted position. They will feel totally relaxed and supported throughout the treatment, and you can take advantage of the full force of gravity to do some of the work for you. Obvious additional benefits include collapsible storage, portability, sturdy construction and a range of accessories such as washable covers in a selection of colourways. Relatively inexpensive, the on-site massage chair is a must for anyone considering frequent use of head massage as a therapeutic tool.

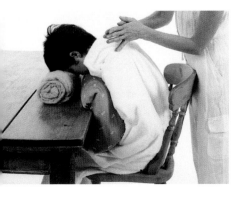

A standard table and chair arrangement, at home or at work, can easily be adapted for delivering 'instant' treatments.

preparing yourself and your partner

Preparing thoroughly for any task you undertake provides a sound basis for all good practice, and helps to fine-tune your mind and body. Taking a little time to pay attention to detail will make your massage treatments much more special and rewarding. Here are a few of the basic principles.

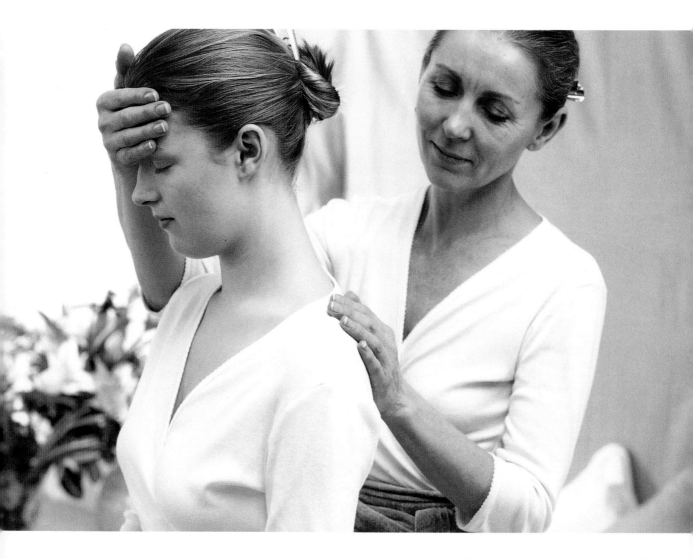

Before you start, make sure that your partner is fully aligned, and that the head is aligned with the base of the spine.

Bathing

Have a warm shower with a body scrub, using a loofah or mitt and unperfumed products. Bear in mind that your choice of deodorant might clash with treatment oils or even be offensive to your partner. Perform the waterfall, the psychic cleansing process, before you start (see page 31).

Hands and nails

Check that your nails are clean, short and polish-free. Wash your hands in warm water as a gesture of respect to your partner's comfort, and ensure that any cuts or grazes are covered with a waterproof dressing.

Hair

Your partner's hair needs to be away from their face and neck during treatment. If their hair is long, tie it back with a cotton head scarf. If your hair is long or bothersome, you have a greater range of options from pinning it up to clipping it back or tying it with hair bands or clips.

Clothing

Wear loose, comfortable clothing which allows your body to breathe and have full range of movement. I recommend natural fabrics and soothing colours to create a relaxing environment.

Safety first

Remind yourself of the basic contra-indications before you start (see the do's and don'ts on pages 28 and 29). Do not be afraid to ask pertinent questions about your partner's health record and current status and discuss with them any stressed, damaged or painful areas in their body. Posture is a key clue so make a point of observing any imbalances or weak areas.

Record book

Keep a note of progressive treatments on the same partner so you have a reference to gauge progress, both theirs and yours.

Final check

Read through the techniques and routines you are going to use during the treatment so that you are clear on your methodology and the movements will flow more easily.

Alignment

Make sure that your partner is fully aligned, that is that the head is aligned with the base of the spine and that their arms and legs are relaxed. Sit or stand squarely onto your partner with your weight evenly distributed and pause to centre yourself before you begin.

Breathing

Before you start, synchronize your breathing patterns. Breathe together in an unforced, natural rhythm so you can connect to your partner's energies.

Finishing touch

End each section and the overall treatment with a loving gesture, such as holding your partner's hand or lightly touching their shoulder.

Refreshment

After the treatment, offer your partner a glass of water to replenish any fluids which may have been lost and to help with the detoxification process which massage promotes.

Reciprocation

Massage can be even more enjoyable if your efforts are reciprocated. This arrangement dispels any feeling of the expert/client relationship, and a healthy balance between unconditional giving and taking will be maintained at the heart of the treatment. Encourage a friend to study the techniques in this book and take it in turns to massage each other. You can compare notes on your treatment successes.

identifying
where to massage

Meridians and the head

The most ancient Eastern medical texts, the Chinese and Japanese in particular, are concerned with the balance of two opposite yet complementary forces, Yin and Yang. Everything in the world, both physical and immaterial, is composed of and affected by these forces – Darkness-Light, Passive-Active, Female-Male, Cold-Hot, Water-Fire, Open-Closed, Soft-Hard. Like everything else in Nature and the wider world, human beings are, in microcosm, subtle mixtures of these qualities. Our bodies, emotions and minds are regulated by the interplay of subtle energy currents known as *ki* or *chi* which flow through channels known as meridians. When the natural balance is disturbed by external forces such as injury, or internally by factors such as stress, therapies like Shiatsu, Reiki and Zone Therapy can readjust the flow of *ki* to restore health. Touch is the universally acknowledged medium by which so many of these treatments are delivered.

Engendering trust

Although the work we have presented in this book takes full account of the principles of such systems, we do not ask you to become experts. A thorough knowledge of Eastern medicine can take years to perfect and is probably only of interest to the professional therapist. Yet a very basic understanding of some of its crucial elements can impart a sense of the subtle and powerful forces involved when you are honoured with the trust of

a loved one or partner who invites you to give a head massage. You will sometimes notice a marked reluctance on the part of the recipient to being touched, an instinct which goes quite deep in most people. Head massage is an intimate treatment: even when you feel you have learnt some useful techniques, please bear in mind that it should only be practised when you are sure you have your partner's full permission.

Flow of ki

Ki or *chi* does not necessarily flow in straight lines as the illustrations opposite indicate. There are node points called *tsubos* where *ki* can most easily be reached and manipulated. For instance, meridians rise to the surface when stretched, hence you will find a number of positions where exact placement of your fingers and thumbs will do the most good. We have included a section (pages 86–97) based on Joseph Corvo's marvellous use of the Zone Therapy approach where you can clearly see the importance of finger massage on predetermined locations.

Despite the demonstrable reality and proven efficacy of Eastern techniques, Western medicine cannot yet conceive of a way to integrate them into an allopathic context. In essence, these energies are non-physical in nature so they have thus far not been amenable to testing and measuring in any meaningful way, in Western scientific terms at least. I can only hope that day will come soon.

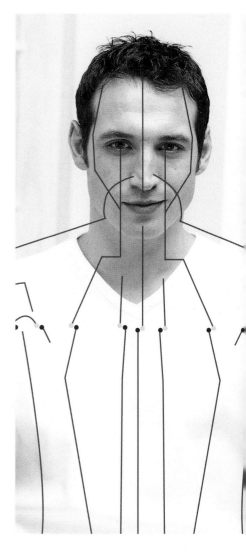

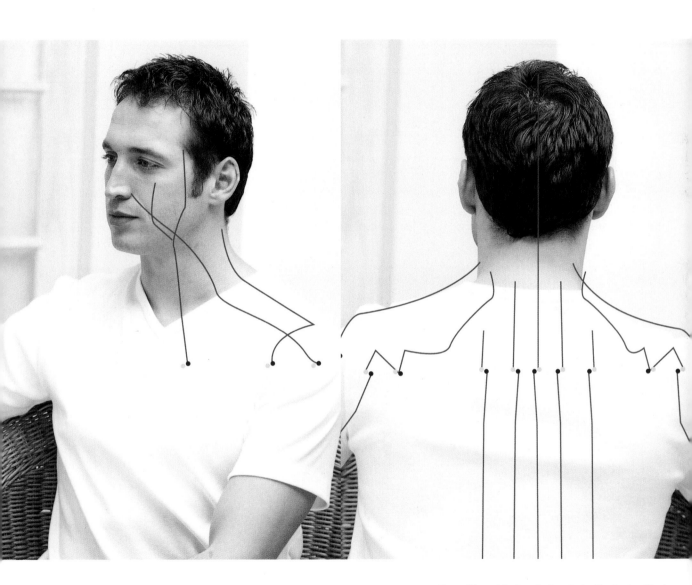

The meridians of the face, front, neck, shoulder, head and back.

natural balance

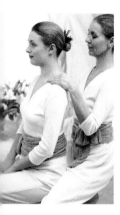

The importance of posture

Being aware of the way you hold your body while working on your partner will help you conserve your energy and ultimately result in a much better treatment. To tone your muscles and ease stiff joints, you can give your body a natural 'work out' with the minimum of effort just by performing everyday movements such as walking, standing, sitting and resting.

When giving a head massage, the golden rules are as follows:
• Keep your weight evenly distributed on the outer edges of your feet so that you don't lean into the insteps.
• Align your body structure, that is the horizontal lines – the right and left sides; and the vertical lines – top and bottom.
• Consciously keep your breath moving in and out in a relaxed, easy rhythm.
• Walk tall and 'grow out' of your joints and muscles, thinking light while feeling grounded.

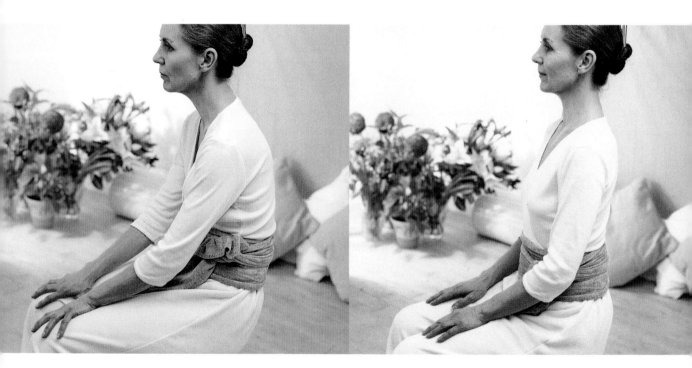

⌃ poor posture

Sinking into your body and collapsing into your emotional centre affects the way you live your whole life. Leaning back you can find your thoughts dwelling in the past while leaning forward you can be grasping at the future. Only when resting in the centre you have the chance to enjoy the present moment.

⌃ sitting correctly

Imagine a book balancing on the crown of your head. Lean your spine slightly forward from the base. Remember that you are aligning not just your body but your mind to the present moment. This basic technique can guard you against future illnesses which are so often caused through physical blocks as the result of poor posture and restrictive clothing.

partner's alignment

Eyes If open, these should be focused just below eye level. If closed, ask your partner to look inwards and visualize *chidakasha*, the inner space known as 'the blackboard of the mind'.

Ears Tops aligned with the lobes to help extend the back of the neck.

Nose In line with the navel to help align the face.

Lips Soft and slightly open to help relax the jaw.

Jaw Relaxed with the tongue away from the roof of the mouth, allowing the breath to flow freely from the nose through to the throat. Make sure that the teeth do not become clenched.

Chin At right angles to the chest to prevent the build-up of tension in the back of the neck.

Chest Open and relaxed to allow movement of the breastbone when breathing.

Shoulders Pulled slightly down and back, contracting the shoulder blades lightly together in order to open up the sternum.

Upper arms Pulled slightly away from the sides of the body (as if there were a small ball of energy in the armpits) to create a sense of space and openness.

Hands Rested lightly on the lap to act as 'damping levers' against the downward pressure of your firmer strokes.

Spine Extended but not rigid, leaning slightly forward from the hips to allow for deeper breathing.

Waist and lower back Muscles here must not be 'overarched' in order to extend the back – there needs to be a sense of flattening this area.

Hips Slightly higher than the knees to prevent the build-up of pressure in the lower back.

Pelvis and pubic bone Tilted slightly forward so the weight, in the seated position, is directly on the anus.

Legs Apart and in line with the hip joints, ensuring that the knees and ankles do not contract, creating unwanted tension in the hips.

Ankles and feet Flat on the floor and grounded, knees over the ball of the feet to create a slight pressure on the 'bubbling spring' (an energy release point), a meridian node on the ball of the foot between the big and second toes.

checklist

masseur's alignment

Head and neck Moving freely with the flow of the massage. Ensure that you do not clench your teeth, purse your lips or frown during the treatment.

Face Passive, with your jaw free and your lips soft, to prevent the build-up of facial tension and the loss of energy and mental focus.

Shoulders Down and back, moving freely with the changing patterns. Go with the rhythm and flow of each movement.

Upper arms Avoid contracting the arms into the body when focusing on percussive movements. Keep your fingers, wrists and elbows relaxed to avoid the build-up of tension in your shoulders and upper back.

Chest Keep the breath flowing freely and avoid collapsing into your emotional centre.

Spine Extended but not rigid, retaining a sense of flexibility. Where possible, the whole of the spine should be in alignment with the crown of the head balanced above the base vertebrae. Do not overarch the spine in an attempt to maintain good posture.

Hips and torso Facing into the working area.

Pelvis Tilted forward slightly so that your seated weight is placed on the anus.

Legs Avoid contracting which will only create tension in the hips and spine. If standing, pull the weight off the knees but do not overextend them. Keep the muscles 'soft'.

Ankles and feet Whenever possible, work in bare feet so that you can be aware of not gripping the floor with your toes and causing tension throughout the whole body.

'A naturally balanced posture treads a fine line between total awareness and total relaxation.'

organic oils, lotions and potions

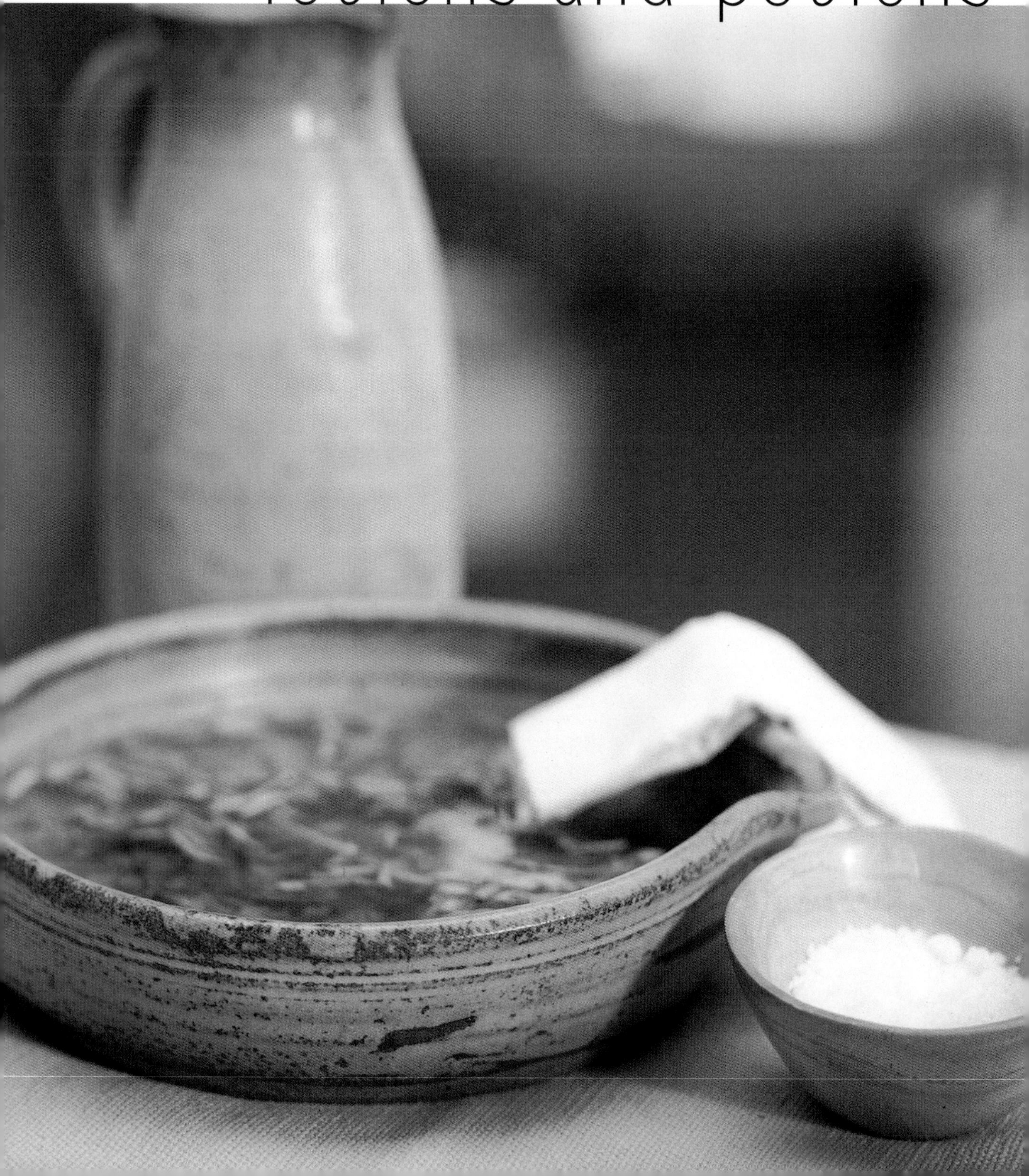

Essential oils

Essential oils are used in aromatherapy (a major therapeutic system in its own right which should not be attempted without prior study). They are obtained from just about every constituent part of plants and trees including roots, stalks, barks, leaves, flowers, blossoms, seeds, nuts, fruits and resins. They all yield valuable active ingredients long known for their therapeutic properties. Except in very rare cases they cannot be used directly on the skin or hair and must be diluted with a carrier or base oil (in a ratio of six drops of essential oil to 10 ml/$^1/_3$ fl oz of carrier oil), before application.

Carrier oils

Carrier or base oils are among the most popular media for all massage treatments. The best, like olive oil, are extracted by the process of cold-pressing. Sunflower, safflower, grapeseed, sesame, sweet almond, avocado and peach nut oil are among the most popular choices. Essential oils are added to carrier oils for aromatherapy treatments.

Lotions

Lotions have a number of advantages, particularly for the beginner. They come premixed at low active-element dosages, they do not run uncontrollably, are unlikely to stain bed linen and are easily absorbed into the skin without leaving an uncomfortably sticky or greasy residue. For your partner's comfort, pre-warm lotions by placing the container in hot water. Do not use lanolin-based lotions as they have a tendency to clog the skin.

Scrubs

Facial and body scrubs are excellent exfoliating media (exfoliation is the removal of dead skin); they are also an important or even essential preparatory beauty treatment. Commercially available or easily homemade from a range of mildly abrasive organic foodstuffs, such as ground rice, oatmeal, pulped nuts, pulses and coconut. Scrubs can reduce the effects of ageing and drying skin (see page 81).

Facial masks

Fuller's Earth is one of the best deep cleansers and makes an excellent base for facial masks. The raw powder, blended to a smooth paste, can be mixed with scented waters such as rose, orange or lavender or made into a rich face pack when mixed with a lotion (see page 82).

Astringents

Astringents are substances that close the pores. Rosewater is an excellent mild natural astringent. It can add that finishing touch to a massage when sprayed or sprinkled onto a fine cloth and placed on the brow (see page 83).

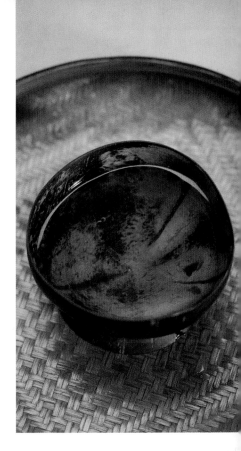

Above: Nature's healing bounty – essential oils.
Opposite: Wat Po's herbal massage mixture.

Compresses

Compresses are very effective at relieving pain and swelling and reducing inflammation. Generally, hot compresses are used to treat chronic pain (backache, fibrositis, rheumatic and arthritic pain, abscesses, earache and toothache) and cold compresses for acute pain, headaches and migraines, and as first-aid for injuries and sprains.

The famous compress known as the Wat Po Herbal Massage Bag consists of casumunar, camphor, kiffer lime and lemongrass. The camphor is dissolved in hot water and cotton or muslin squares are thoroughly soaked in the mixture. These are then wrapped around the dried medicinal herbs and tied into bags. They are left to steam periodically when they are not being applied to the affected area.

safe and effective home treatments

Do not be put off by the guidelines below. Head massage is perfectly safe for most people in moderate health and under most circumstances. In the words of Florence Nightingale: 'Nature alone cures . . . what has to be done . . . is to put the person in the best condition for Nature to act upon.'

Body assessment

Acute observation of all the factors and conditions outlined below will help your head massage treatments to be not only more effective but also safer. Generally, note the following factors which give clues to the type of treatment which is most appropriate for your partner. Professional practitioners, as a matter of course, will request and require the answers to most of these questions before it is safe to use any aromatherapy oils or lotions with active essential ingredients. If you have any reservations about whether to treat anyone suffering from a debilitating medical condition, please encourage them to get advice from their doctor before your treatment.

Does your partner suffer any of the following conditions?

Dietary problems Diabetes, over- or underweight, anorexia, bulimia, ulcers, colitis, constipation, flatulence, diahorrea, indigestion
Muscle tone and texture Tense, relaxed, contracted, tender, unconditioned
Skin type Very dry, very oily, sensitive, cracked, irritated, inflamed, blotchy
Sluggish or poor circulation
Spinal problems Curved or distorted, prolapsed disk or spondylosis
Joint problems Stiff, inflamed, painful, inflexible, swollen.

Medication

Take into account any medication or homeopathic remedies your partner may be taking or any conditions such as epilepsy which could appear or be triggered merely by the actions of your massage or the effects of such complete relaxation.

Stress release

Be prepared for your partner to exhibit all kinds of stress release. These may include a variety of reactions from crying to laughing, coughing, sighing, moaning or groaning, even passing wind. Reassure them that it is perfectly normal and is, in itself, a natural healing response.

Time

Do give yourself plenty of time to accomplish your treatment and allow your partner to rest afterwards in order to enjoy the effects of your labours.

Rehydration

Apart from being a pleasant social end to your treatment, it is essential to rehydrate the skin and body with a glass of water. This will help to remove the toxins released by your massage. A small slice of citrus fruit may be added for taste.

Please take the time to read this section carefully and observe its guidelines to the letter until your own skills, intuition and knowledge of the body's systems develop enough for you to know how and when to make significant exceptions.

There are, of course, a number of contra-indications to treatment, some of which might be obvious, others less so. You bear an important responsibility when you interact with another's physical being and bioenergetic energies. Again, a few well-chosen questions will reveal important information which you must use to evaluate whether or not to engage in a head massage treatment. The key ones are listed here.

Acupuncture

Do not offer a treatment to anyone who has had an acupuncture treatment on the same day. Their energies will already be redefining their flow and any treatment you offer may interfere with this newly adjusting balance.

Alcohol

It is not advisable to give a massage to anyone with substantial amounts of alcohol in their bloodstream.

Back problems

These include prolapsed disks, damaged vertebrae, spinal injury and whiplash. In cases other than muscle strain, advise your partner to seek the advice and treatment of a specialist such as an osteopath, chiropractor or physiotherapist before giving a massage.

Bathing

Make sure that your partner only has a warm shower, rather than a hot bath or shower, before a treatment. Expanded and loose muscles can easily be overstretched or overworked, leading to potential future problems.

Blood pressure

Give a lighter touch for anyone suffering high blood pressure and a firmer touch for those with low blood pressure.

Cancer

Give only gentle facial treatments or head wrappings with essential oils in such cases.

Driving and using machinery

Advise your partner not to drive or operate heavy machinery if they feel at all drowsy after their massage.

Eating

Head massage can be performed at any time other than immediately after eating. Allow at least half an hour after a light meal and at least an hour after a particularly heavy one.

Skin conditions

Do not massage over open wounds, cuts, swellings, sprains, boils, carbuncles, septic conditions, weeping eczema, psoriasis, shingles or other infections.

Above all, be sensible. Do not undertake massage of anyone you know has a medical condition with which you are either not conversant or knowledgeable or do not have their doctor's or therapist's permission. This might well include conditions such as epilepsy, schizophrenia, Down's Syndrome, deep depression, migraines, meningitis, diabetes, thrombosis, embolism or an advanced heart condition, fainting or dizzy spells.

'Treat the ones you can and leave the ones you can't.' On the rare occasions I have felt it sensible to refuse treatment I have only been appreciated for my honesty and professionalism.

energetic cleansing

Creating a sacred inner space

Anyone who has practised massage in its many forms knows that it is more than merely a physical therapy. Whenever human beings interact there is a subtle flow and exchange of energies. Whether this understanding or knowledge is part of your personal belief system, you should understand that it is a reality to many people, possibly including the partner you are planning to massage. If you deem your gift of time and skills to be worthwhile to others, then you must be sensitive to the potential harm as well as the benefits within your energetic being. I urge you to discover for yourself the true reality behind the merely physical.

'Centring' is an important way of focusing your energy into a point from which it can easily be channelled into the task at hand – your forthcoming head massage treatment. It is a state of metaphysical equilibrium. Your centre is known as the *Hara*, the Japanese word for belly or abdomen. The Chinese refer to it as *Tan t'ien* and the Yogic/Tantric tradition as *Manipura chakra*. Located a few inches below the navel, it is associated with the digestive fire, the seat of one's emotional life; it is your centre of gravity – the nucleus of your physical being.

Locating and channelling your personal energy through the *Hara* means that your treatment requires less muscle power, and you can work for longer, with less energy depletion and with little or no emotional drain. Before any touch

therapy, spend a few minutes centring yourself. Sit cross-legged on a chair or the floor (with a folded blanket under the hips if necessary). Ensure that your hips are slightly higher than your knees. Physically align the whole spine and rest the backs of your hands on your knees, thumbs holding the forefingers in place, the other fingers curling naturally. Close your eyes and focus your attention on the third eye (*Ajna chakra*). Connect your

Centring is a vital prerequisite of any healing practice.

base vertebrae squarely onto the chair or floor, allowing the spine to 'float' upwards. Observe the natural flow of your breath, letting it find its own rhythm. Inhale. Imagine filling your *Hara* with strength and energy from the earth. Feel the upward flow of energy into the *Hara*

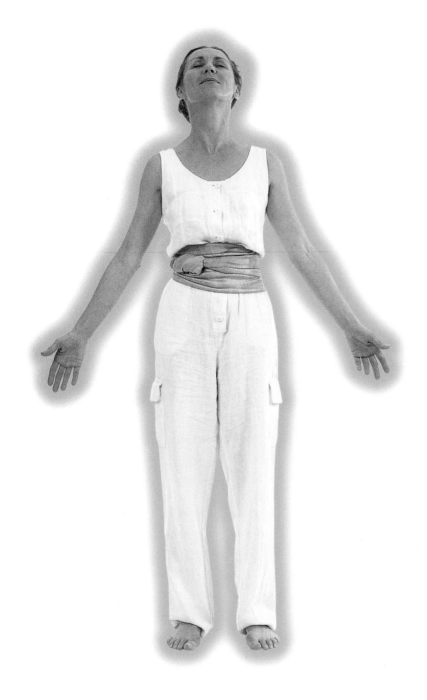

The waterfall is one of the most useful psychic cleansing techniques.

The waterfall

The waterfall, and similar variations, is a psychic cleansing technique best practised before any healing interaction with another person. It may be performed as a ritual during a pre-session shower or as a visualization if showering is not possible.

Imagine you are standing beneath a crystal-clear waterfall. Its life-giving and refreshing waters cleanse you of your daily travails, petty concerns and any negativities in your mental attitude. The water pools and collects around your feet and flows out into the natural world where it is purified and reintegrated into the flow of all Mother Nature.

The waterfall may also be practised after a head massage session and will also cleanse your psychic body of any impurities, negativities, concerns or otherwise clinging remnants of your treatment. It is vital that your partner's mental state and concerns do not remain with you after the session. Wash them all away.

Salt has long been known for its alchemical efficacy in absorbing negative energies. Some therapists place a small bowl of salt crystals near their working area. During a treatment they 'flick' or discharge 'dirty' or excess energies into this primal element. Salt is cleansed by prolonged exposure to sunlight (although I would not recommend using it on your food after that!).

After any session of head massage therapy it is important to cleanse oneself. This has a double benefit: it is a psychic letting go of a temporary attachment to your partner's energy body, their worries and concerns, and also of your attachment to the outcome of your work. All true healing is unconditional. Run your hands and wrists under fresh, flowing water after any treatment. Do this psychically with the waterfall visualization if facilities are not available.

and along your arms and down through your fingers. Continue until you feel ready to do the treatment. I offer my personal mantra – a thought I hold in my mind while performing any treatment: 'There is a healing light shining in the centre of my being.'

'Smudging' is one of the better-known of the Native American cleansing techniques. The herb sage, a highly aromatic plant, is dried and tied into bundles. Prior to utilizing any space for healing or sacred purposes, a little of the herb is then burned to 'cleanse' both the physical and psychic. Traditionally an eagle's feather is used to waft the smoke around the room and the bodies of both healer and recipient.

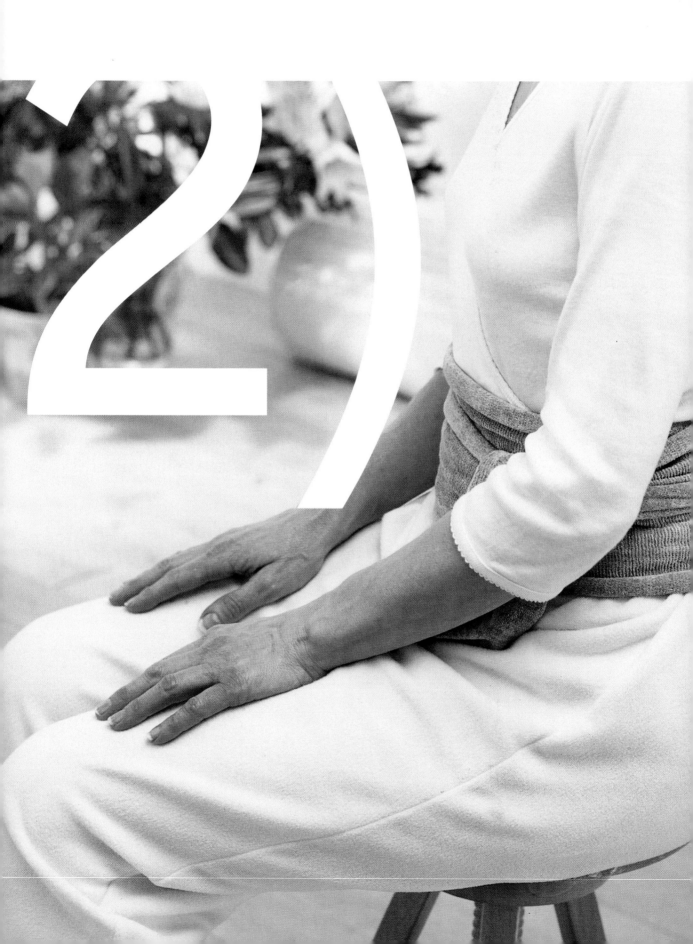

basic routines

Gentle friction techniques

The gentle friction techniques are warming, soothing and calming. They can be used on almost anybody and at any time (see contra-indications on page 29 for exceptions) without requiring lubricants. Being slow and rhythmical, they are not only immensely comforting to the recipient, but also provide the masseur with a useful pause for reflection and preparation between techniques. Even the sound they make as they are applied can reinforce their calming and soothing effect.

basic techniques

smoothing

The smoothing technique can be used over the head, hair, face, neck, shoulders and back and usually heralds the beginning or end of a technique or sequence. It performs an essential muscle-warming function – a necessary prelude to more vigorous techniques – and is an effective muscle relaxant afterwards. Its stronger action towards the heart assists the return of venous blood, and its lighter application away from it removes energetic 'impurities'.

interlacing

Interlacing is a slightly more powerful version of the smoothing technique. It is, perhaps, more suitable for men with a well-developed musculature who often appreciate a more definite pressure. Placing the mother hand on top of the working one and interlacing the fingers provides a broad platform for the larger body areas. The natural pattern of application is either a small or large figure of eight.

scrubbing

Less expansive and more localized than the smoothing and interlacing techniques, scrubbing allows you to work into the smaller contours of the body. Because of its more rapid application, it has a stronger localized warming effect. The technique entails making a soft claw of your working hand, then 'scrubbing' the flat of your nails, in small circular movements, over the muscle areas of the shoulders, back and upper arms. Scrubbing should only be applied up to the level of your partner's preference or tolerance.

Percussive techniques

Although the full range of a masseur's percussive techniques usually include pummelling and plucking, they are not particularly appropriate for the subject of this book, the more sensitive head massage. The main value of percussion is to stimulate the soft tissue areas, tone the skin and improve circulation. Largely reserved for the heavily muscled areas such as the trapezius (the yoke across the shoulders) and the upper arms, I have graded the three techniques in their order of speed and pressure. The key to all of them is to keep the hands relaxed and the wrists loose. I recommend that novices practise them on their own thighs which, in any case, is a wonderful antidote to cellulite! Shake your hands well before you start (to avoid cramp) and do not use the technique directly on the spinal column.

'MOTHER' AND 'WORKING' HANDS

Throughout the book, reference will be made to the 'mother' and 'working' hands. When you are massaging, your less dominant hand is simply used to maintain an energetic and comforting connection with your partner. Known as the 'mother' hand, it is largely static and supportive, and is used to 'listen' for reactions to your treatments. The 'working' hand, whether left or right by preference, is simply the more active agent.

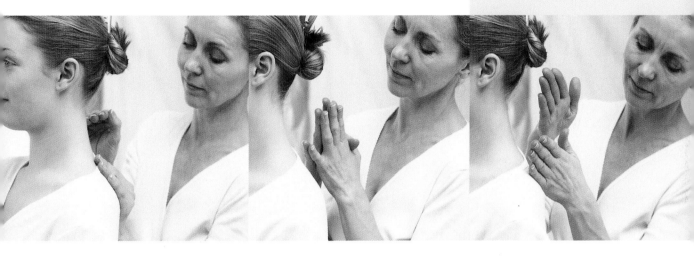

cupping

The cupping technique is a rapid sequence of alternate drumming strokes formed by your cupped hands trapping air against the skin. Particularly when performed directly on the skin, rather than through clothing, its release makes a loud sucking sound. Arch your hands at the knuckles, keeping your fingers straight, and rapidly and alternately 'cup' the area you are working on. Work methodically, paying attention to your partner's comfort. Thirty seconds or so should suffice for most treatments. Smooth off with one of the gentle friction techniques.

clicking

Slightly stronger than the cupping technique, the 'clicking' sound is produced by the splayed fingers which have the damping effect of a spring. Lightly press your palms together, overlapping the thumbs and slightly splaying the fingers. Beat downwards with the edge of the little fingers, allowing the other fingers to close together. With a timed beat of three quick movements, lift off, pause, then repeat over the chosen muscle area. With care, clicking can even be performed lightly over the head. Smooth off with one of the gentle friction techniques.

hacking

The strongest of the percussion techniques, hacking is particularly useful and necessary for the well-muscled male torso. Adopting what many comically term the 'karate chop' form with thumbs relaxed and fingers together, alternatively beat the edges of your fingers and hands over any heavily muscled areas. Keep your hands and shoulders relaxed. This seemingly violent movement must be matched to the capability and tolerance of your partner. Performed correctly it is a most pleasant experience. Smooth off with one of the gentle friction techniques.

Stretching and aligning

The stretching and aligning techniques outlined below are very gentle postural fine-tunings of the body shape and are not to be considered a substitute for the kind of professional manipulation offered by osteopaths, chiropractors and physiotherapists. However, a sensitive fine-tuning of your partner's postural alignment is a key element in re-educating poor posture, so often the cause of chronic pain, muscular distress and a range of common conditions such as headaches, migraines and depression. If you discover serious misalignment, please recommend professional consultation. On no account practise any of the stretching and aligning techniques on anyone you know to have suffered a whiplash injury, or who has an observed or reported spinal misalignment. These techniques should ideally be performed with your partner in a sitting or standing position. Alternatively, sit your partner on the floor, and kneel and support their back with your raised knee and thigh. Performed correctly and sensitively, these techniques greatly ease tension from the neck and spine.

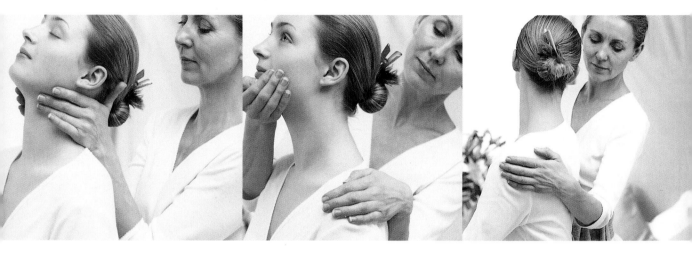

traction

Using one of the gentle friction techniques, first warm and relax the muscles of the neck and shoulders. Sit or stand squarely behind your partner, roughly half a head higher. Cradle their head in your hands, with your palms supporting the base of the skull and your fingers under the jawline. Take the weight of their head in your hands, lifting slightly as you bring your forearms between the shoulder blades and either side of the spine. Gently ease the head back using the forearms as both support and lever. Hold for two or three breaths, ease back to the central starting position and repeat slowly three times.

tilting

Stand or sit to one side of your partner. Place your working hand under your partner's chin for support, with your opposite forearm resting lightly on the trapezius muscle. Initially place the mother hand on the other shoulder. As you slowly tilt the head back, bring the mother hand forearm underneath the neck to support the movement. Gently ease the head backwards and forwards with the support of the working hand and forearm. Ensure that your partner remains in postural alignment and does not arch the lower back to accommodate the stretch. Repeat the movements from three to six times.

twisting

Keeping the mother hand and forearm in place across the back of the shoulders, pull back the nearest shoulder, gently twisting the upper body towards you. Ask your partner to turn their head in the same direction and 'go with the movement'. If the spine is stiff, allow just the head to move naturally. Relax the movement and allow the body to return to its front-facing position. Repeat three times. Shift your position and repeat the technique on the other side of the body, again three times.

Easing and comforting

This next set of techniques I think of as easing and comforting movements, and I may use them at any time during a massage session. Light and rhythmical, they are easy to learn as well as being a pleasurable boon to the recipient and a great workout for the masseur's hands. I have included the cradling technique, partly to illustrate the supportive and comforting nature of closeness and touch so often denied legitimate expression for some people. At times the process of massage can release long-suppressed tensions and withheld emotional pain. Do not be afraid to respond in a loving and nurturing way at these crucial moments. You will know when it is fitting and appropriate. The picture of the cradling technique here captures a delightfully precious interlude with my darling daughter, Emily.

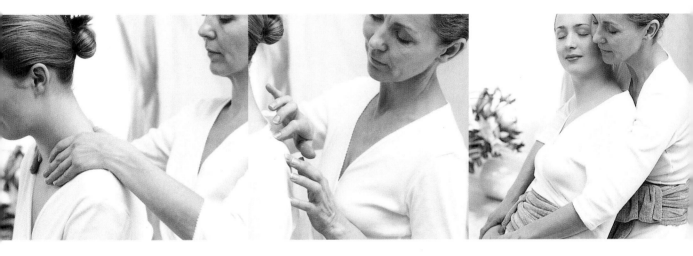

circling

Position your hands lightly on the shoulders on either side of the neck. Place the thumbs on the muscles on either side of the spine as far down as you can reach. Starting with an inward and upward circle, use the full pressure of the thumbs to make circling movements on the often-tight trapezius muscles between the shoulder blades. Start with large circles (right thumb clockwise, left thumb anticlockwise) on the area closest to the shoulder blade. You can progress the circling up the back and onto either side of the neck, adapting the hand positions to allow a natural flow of movements.

piano walking

Imagine you are playing the piano on the trapezius and other soft muscle areas. The pressure you apply will depend on your personal strength, the comfort/pleasure feedback you get from your partner, and your intuition of the moment. The technique, suitably modified in pressure, can be used to great effect over the skull and along the neck. Pressure is applied from the tips of the fingers and should only be attempted if the nails are short enough not to indent the skin too much. Smooth off with interlaced fingers.

cradling

This is a wonderful finishing touch or, if appropriate, it can be introduced during the treatment if your partner needs more emotional support. Cradle their body close to yours and gently rock from side to side or round in small circles.

Detoxifying techniques

The lymphatic system helps to maintain the correct fluid balance in the tissues and the blood, defends against disease and removes cellular waste products. Lymph, a milky fluid derived from the blood, circulates around the body in a network of tiny vessels, clusters of which are located in the neck, armpits, groin, knees and the middle of the torso. The detoxifying massage techniques described below act like a pump to stimulate the flow of lymphatic fluids, helping them to remove waste products such as lactic acid from the bloodstream.

As with the stretching and aligning techniques, do not perform any of these movements on anyone you know to have suffered a whiplash injury or to have an observed or reported spinal misalignment.

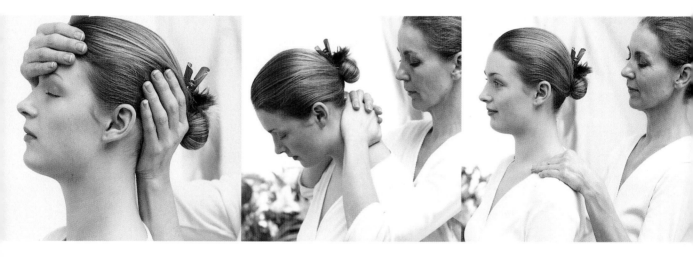

pressing

Cradle your partner's brow with your supporting or mother hand and tilt the head slightly forward at first. Slowly and firmly press the heel of your working hand up the line of the neck muscles on one side of the neck to the base of the skull. Hold for 3–4 seconds, repeating the movement up the other side of the neck and holding for the same length of time.

heel squeezing

Ask your partner to relax their head and upper torso, tilting it slightly forward. Closely and firmly interlace your fingers and place them over the back of the neck. Using gentle but insistent leverage, squeeze the heels of the hands together, applying reasonable pressure on the neck muscles. Hold for 2–3 seconds and gently release the pressure. Repeat the sequence two or three times.

squeezing and lifting

Gently squeeze and lift the top of the trapezius muscle, starting at the end nearest the shoulder joint, using the strength of the thumbs, forefingers and middle fingers. Squeeze, lift and hold for 2–3 seconds. Release and move your working hand a little closer to the neck and repeat until the whole muscle has been worked on. Smooth across the working area (and down the arms if you like) to finish and provide a relaxing comfort stroke.

Variation *Use the pads of your working fingers instead of the heel of your hand. This gives a slightly stronger massage for those with very stiff muscles.*

Variation *The heel squeezing technique can also be used to apply a good level of pressure over the trapezius muscles and the upper arms, if required. Smooth off to finish.*

Stimulating and embodying techniques

Clearly the pictures on this page illustrate the effectiveness of the techniques on long hair. Of course, many people have either short hair or none at all. This is no problem. The aim and benefit of these techniques are to stimulate the scalp which can be worked upon directly. Except during a vigorous hair wash, the scalp is seldom exercised and often suffers poor blood circulation and builds up dry, scaly skin (dandruff); and this can even lead to mental tiredness and apathy. Although it might seem the very last thing one would wish to do while suffering a stress-induced headache, tugging and pulling at the hair close to the scalp can often provide instant relief. Alternatively, vigorous circling of the fingertips to move the scalp over the skull will accomplish a similar result.

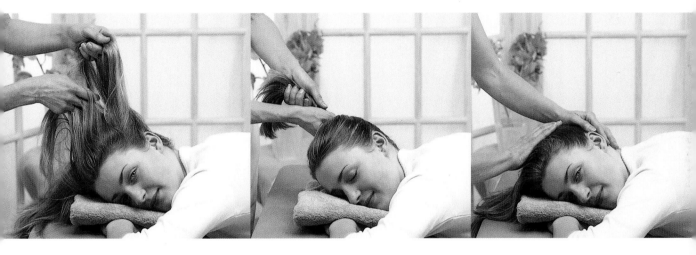

lifting and lightening

Lie your partner face down on a made-up bed, massage couch or on-site massage chair. Comb through the hair, rubbing closely into the scalp with your fingertips. Working on short hair can be equally beneficial, if not as expansive. Comb through to the ends of the hair, allowing it to trickle through your fingers. Repeat all over the scalp to give a sense of lightness.

pulling the hair

Twist the hair into a knot and gently pull with your working hand close to the scalp. Repeat two or three times.

stroking

Stroke over the hair (or head), starting at the base of the neck or even lower, between the shoulder blades. Repeat no more than ten times, turning the head to repeat on the other side.

Variation *Brush the scalp and hair with a natural bristle brush, pulling the hair up and away from the back of the neck.*

Variation *Pull the hair in small clumps close to the scalp and rotate the hair to move the scalp muscles. This relieves tension headaches.*

hi-ki basic routine

I have illustrated this routine with the recipient lying down which is probably the easiest position for this type of massage. Alternatively, stand with your partner sitting on a stool or chair, ensuring that their head is at waist height, or sit with your partner on a cushion in front of you, cradled by your body. If you choose the prone position (lying down), support their neck with a rolled hand towel for the first half of the session.

This routine encapsulates all of the fundamental strokes you will use in most head massage. Work on a clean face, free of any make-up. Apply a few drops of carrier oil or a rich, non-scented massage lotion (available from many high street stores) onto your fingertips before working it in with the pattern of the movements.

⋀ 1) cradling the head

Gently cradle your hands on either side of your partner's head, with your fingertips touching the tops of their ears. Pause for a minute to centre yourself and to give your partner a chance to become accustomed to your touch.

Caution: Make sure your partner does not wear contact lenses during the treatment.

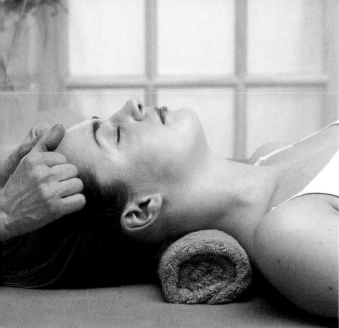

≪ 2) smoothing the brow

Mentally divide the forehead into horizontal strips, about 1 cm (½ in) wide. Starting with the outer edges of your thumbs at the centre of the forehead (just below the widow's peak), glide outwards along the topmost section using moderate pressure. Continue all the way down to the temples and end with a gentle single circle about 1 cm (½ in) wide.

Return to the centre of the forehead and begin the next strip. Repeat until the whole forehead has been smoothed, ending in a single circle each time.

3) circling the temples ≫

Still using the outer edges of your thumbs, circle around the temples (the small hollows on either side of the eyes) in a clockwise direction away from your working position. Repeat six times, keeping your touch very light.

Pause for a few seconds and gently lift off to the next step.

benefit

This step can be very useful in easing tension headaches and mental distress, and invokes a feeling of calmness and inner serenity.

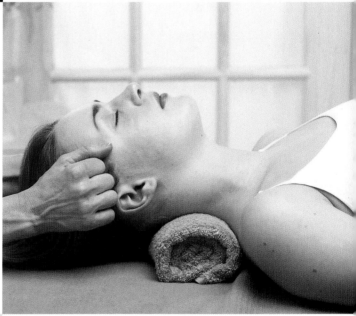

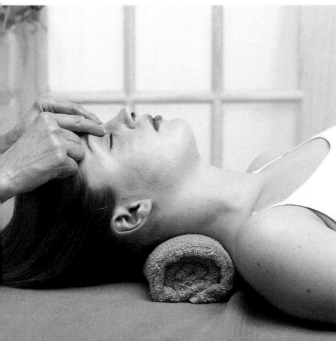

≪ 4) pinching the nasal bone

Gently press your forefingers against the bridge of the nose and hold for a few seconds.

Ease both forefingers along against the bony rims of the eye sockets where the nose joins the eyes. Press a little more firmly for a few seconds.

Lift your fingers and move them 1 cm (½ in) along the upper half of each rim. Press, hold and release.

Continue the pressing movements in increments of about 1 cm (½ in) along the eye sockets to the point furthest from the nose.

Return to the starting position and repeat the press-hold-release sequence along the rim of the eye socket beneath the eyeball.

As a finishing touch, gently press one forefinger onto the bridge of the nose, pause and release.

hi-ki basic routine

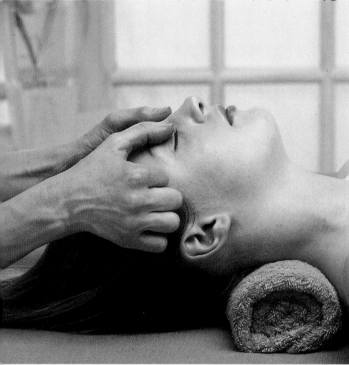

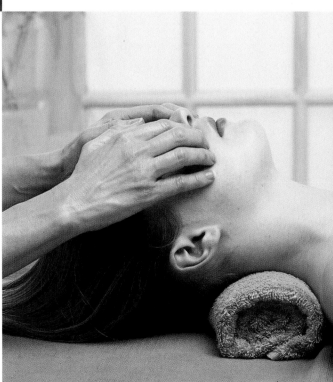

≪ 5) smoothing the eyelids

Starting beside the nose in the corner of the eye, very slowly and lightly run the pads of both thumbs across the closed eyelids using the minimum of pressure (as if trying to straighten the creases in the skin). Repeat three times.

As a finishing touch, gently press the outer edge of the eyelid, pause and release before moving on to the next step.

benefit
_____

Soothes tired eyes.

6) pressing the cheekbones ≫

Place the tips of the forefingers and index fingers on either side of the nose, immediately below the starting position of the last step, that is, the corner of the eye socket.

Pressing firmly, draw the tips of these fingers around the lower edges of the cheekbones and up towards the ears.

Circle the temple once with the fingertips.

Repeat the stroke, ending with another circle.

As a finishing touch, gently press the temple with the index finger, pause and lift the hands off before moving to the next step.

Variation *Repeat the step with tiny circles from the sides of the nose to the temple.*

benefit
_____

Relieves facial tensions.

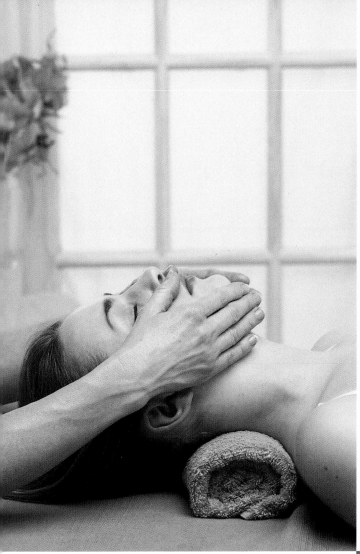

≪ 7) smoothing the lips

For this step, you need to imagine the lower half of the face divided into three horizontal bands: above the lips, the lips themselves, and below the lower lips.

Cupping the jaw, place your thumbs above the upper lip.

Smooth outwards and slightly upward onto the cheeks and towards the temples, ending with a small circle. Repeat three times.

Repeat the sequence across the lips themselves and then under the lower lips, always ending with a circle at the temple.

As a finishing touch, gently press the temples with the index finger, pause and lift the hands off to move onto the next step.

8) smoothing the chin and jaw ≫

With the hands cupping the jaw, firmly pinch the flesh of the chin between forefingers and thumbs.

Firmly smooth along the line of the jaw, finishing with six small circular movements in the 'hinge' just below the earlobes. Use the circular repetitions of the forefingers and index fingers to locate and firmly work the area. The thumbs, resting lightly on the temples, will be your anchor points.

As a finishing touch, lightly press the heels of the hands into the jaw hinges.

benefit

Prevents and relieves neuralgia, earache and headaches.

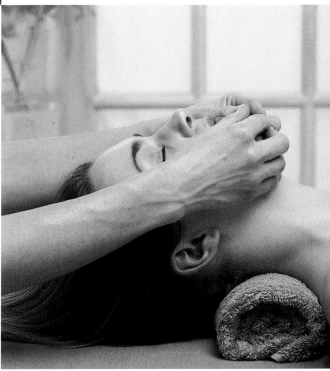

hi-ki basic routine

9) pressing behind the ear »

Working on one ear at a time, ease the head slightly to one side. Gently smooth up the crease behind the ear from the lobe to the top using the tips of your fingers. Repeat three times.

Centralize the head and ease it over to the opposite side. Repeat the step on the other ear.

benefit

Can relieve earache.

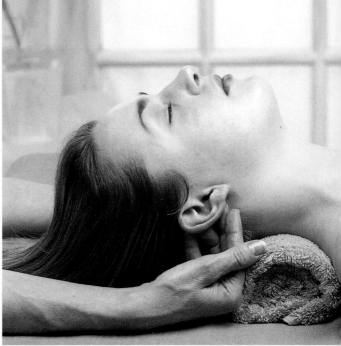

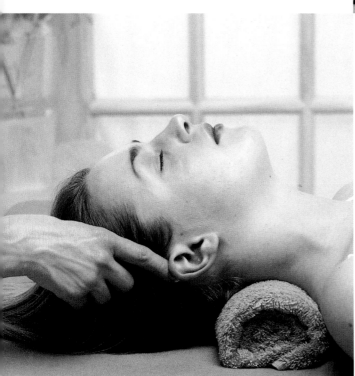

« 10) pressing above the ear

Working on one ear at a time, ease the head slightly to one side. Gently run the length of your forefinger back and forth several times in the 'V' formed by the topmost part of the ear and the head.

Centralize the head and ease it over to the opposite side. Repeat the step on the other ear.

benefit

Can relieve earache.

11) pinching the outer edge of the ear »

Lightly pinch the outer edges of the ears between the thumbs and forefingers, starting at the very top of the ear, and work down towards the lobe.

Pinch and pull the lobe down and hold for two to three seconds. Repeat two or three times.

As a finishing touch, rub the palms of your hands together until they are really warm, then cup them lightly over your partner's ears. Hold for a few breaths, allowing the heat to penetrate.

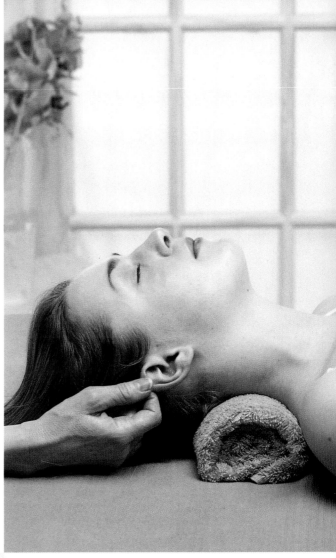

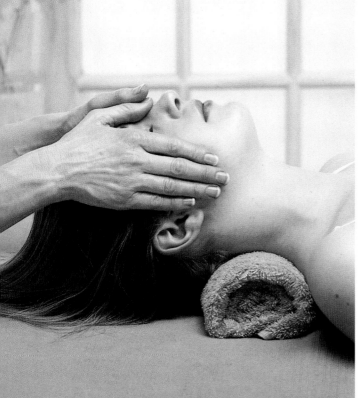

« 12) smoothing the face

Gently cross the thumbs on the tip of the nose and rest the hands over the face, covering the eyes.

Hold for a few breaths and slowly draw the hands upwards, thumbs pressing lightly into the nose, then the forehead. Imagine smoothing away all the lines of worry, stress and strain.

Smooth down the sides to the temples, gently circling in an anti-clockwise direction towards your body.

As a finishing touch, gently press the outer edges of your thumbs into the temples, pause and release.

hi-ki basic routine

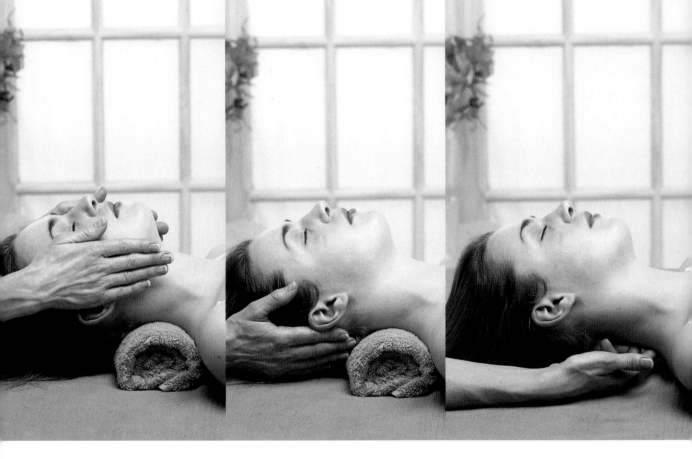

⌃ 13) pressing and circling the temples and cheeks

Hold the temples in the palms of your hands for 5–10 seconds. Using the heels of your hands and a fairly firm pressure, move the temples in clockwise circles away from your body, six times.

Continuing with the circular flow, move down over the cheekbones onto the cheeks, circling another six times to stimulate the whole face.

⌃ 14) pressing the head

Slide your hands gently over the ears and tuck them behind the ears, resting on the massage surface. Press and hold for 5–10 seconds, release slightly and repeat the pressure/release sequence three times.

benefit

Can help to relieve pressure headaches.

⌃ 15) piano walking

Remove the towel roll from behind the neck.

Support your partner's head with your mother hand. Piano-walk the fingers of your working hand into the back of the neck and shoulders to break up any areas of tension. Massage only on the side of the working hand.

Swap hand positions to treat the other side of the neck and shoulders.

Allow approximately 30 seconds for each side, revisiting the site of any especially tense areas or those favoured by your partner.

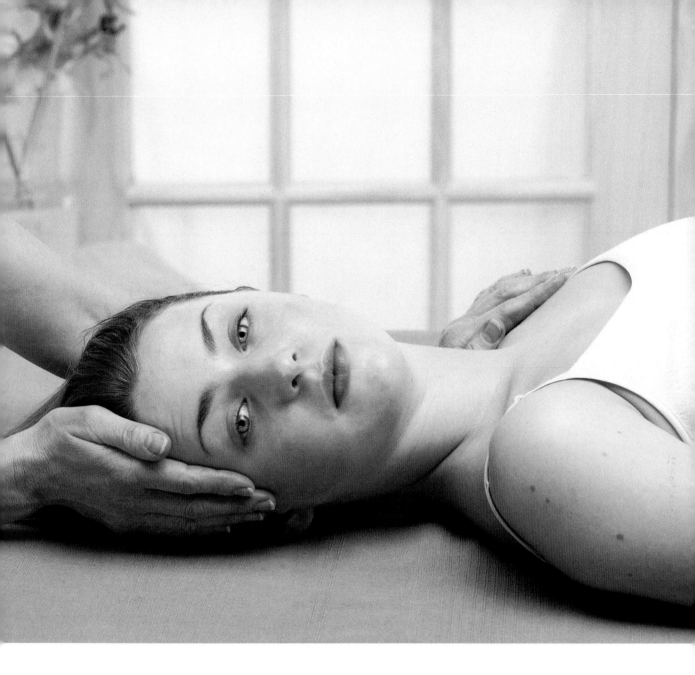

仌 16) easing the neck and shoulders

Turn your partner's head to one side, supporting it with your working hand.

Press the opposite shoulder into the bed with your mother hand and hold for 2–3 seconds. Release and repeat three times.

Turn your partner's head to the opposite side, supporting it with your mother hand.

Press the opposite shoulder into the bed with your working hand and hold for 2–3 seconds. Release and repeat three times.

Variation *From the starting position of pressing the shoulder down, smooth over the shoulder and upper arm, continuing under the shoulder and along the trapezius muscle and up onto the neck in a continuous, large, circular movement. Repeat two or three times on each side.*

benefit

Greatly relieves neck and shoulder tension, particularly after a long period of driving.

hi-ki basic routine

⩘ 17) pressing the chest

Place your hands over the shoulders, with the heels against the trapezius muscle and the fingers resting on the upper part of the chest, forming a triangle.

Press down firmly and hold for 5–10 seconds. Release and repeat three times.

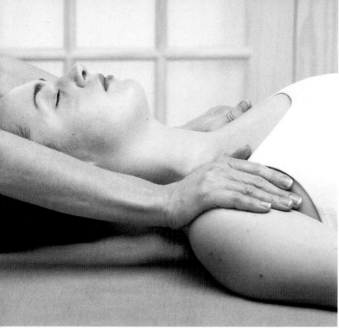

≪ 18) pressing the shoulders

Smooth outwards, across the chest, resting the hands on the shoulders and upper arms. Press firmly down into the massage surface to help open the upper chest.

Release slightly and repeat the movement three times.

19) pushing the shoulders ≫

Rest your hands over the tops of the shoulders and push them down in the direction of the feet with a firm and steady pressure. Hold for 5–10 seconds.

Release slightly and repeat the movement three times.

benefit

As a sequence, steps 17, 18 and 19 are an excellent antidote to rounded shoulders and poor postural alignment.

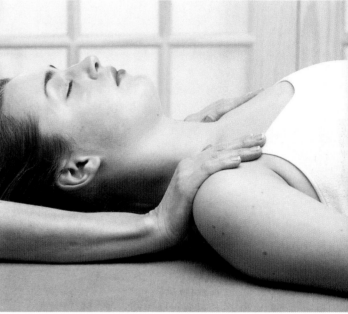

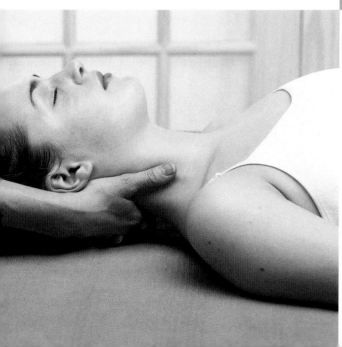

≪ 20) pulling the neck

Slip your hands under the back of the neck, interlacing the fingers fully. Slowly and gently ease and pull the neck towards you, using the power of the clasped hands to exert a gentle but consistent pressure against the base of the skull.

Release slightly and repeat the pulling movement three times.

hi-ki basic routine

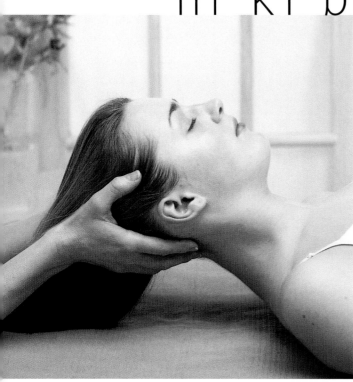

« 21) lifting and tilting the head

Slide your hands back from the position in the previous step to cradle the back of the skull in the palm of your hands, with your fingertips on the muscles at the base.

Moving very slowly and gently, lift and tilt the chin towards the chest. Do not force the action – the limit of your partner's stretch should be obvious.

Lower the head slowly and gently and repeat the movement three times.

As a finishing touch, gently cradle the resting head between your palms and rock slightly from side to side two or three times.

Caution: The human adult head can weigh as much as 7 kg (16 lb). Be sure you have a well-supported stance and give full confidence at all times to your partner.

22) smoothing the neck and hair »

Continuing from the previous step, place your mother hand on the upper part of the forehead (to provide support and stability) and the working hand under the back of the neck, below the skull.

Pull your working hand towards you, elongating the neck with a gentle insistence, and allow it to smooth under the back of the skull until you can grasp the hair at the crown of the head. Even if your partner has short hair you can still make the same movement. Perform only once very slowly.

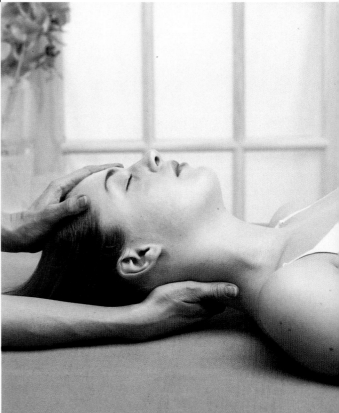

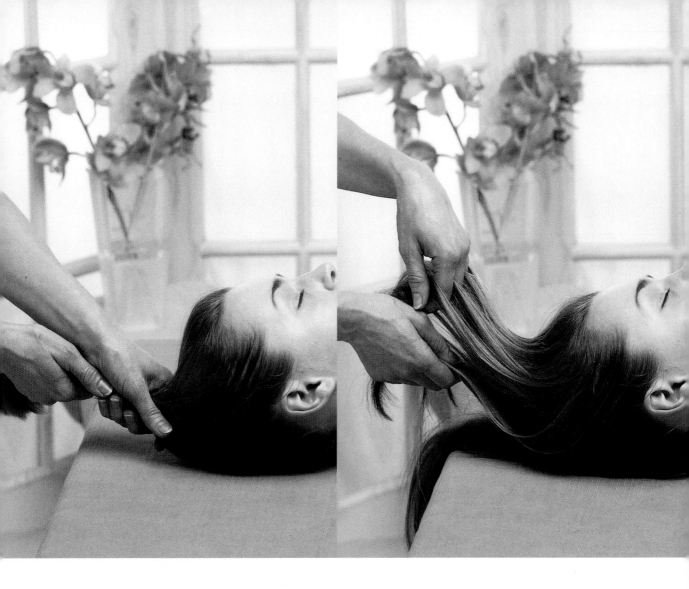

⩘ 23) gathering and pulling the hair

Draw the hair upwards towards the crown. If the hair is short, simply smooth backwards and upwards.

Twist the hair into a knot and hold closely near the skull. Gently pull, to help release any pressure in the head. Unravel the hair and gently smooth back into place.

If the hair is short, take small amounts of hair between your thumb and the side of your forefinger, twisting it to get a grip. Pull, hold and release, working in various places across the head. If the hair is too short to do this, or absent altogether, then press various parts of the scalp with your middle finger and rotate firmly with a circular motion.

As a finishing touch, trace the hair's natural flowing lines with your fingertips.

benefit

Playful sporting with the hair has, from time immemorial, been a recognized remedy for mild headaches.

⩘ 24) lifting and lightening

Lightly 'comb' the scalp, allowing the hair to lift and trickle through your fingers. The movements are just as soothing and beneficial to someone with short hair.

Keep repeating the process to give a sense of space and lightness.

Variation *The hair can be lightly plaited and unplaited if it is long enough. Lightly comb through the hair with the fingertips so that it flows away from the head.*

hi-ki basic routine

⌃ 25) turning the head

Lightly cup the hands over your partner's ears and turn the head to one side until your hand is lying on the massage surface. Hold for 5–10 seconds.

Return the head to the centre line, pausing slightly, then turn to the opposite side. Again, hold for 5–10 seconds before returning to the centre.

⌃ 26) circling the neck

Resting the mother hand on one shoulder, cradle the neck, up to the base of the skull, in the palm of your working hand.

Gently ease the head towards the mother hand as far as is comfortable for your partner. Then smooth the back of the neck, with the whole of your hand, two or three times in a clockwise direction towards your body. This will ease out accumulated neck tension.

Return the head to the centre line, swap hand positions and ease the head in the opposite direction. Again, smooth the neck with clockwise movements before returning the head to the centre line.

⌃ 27) oiling the third eye

Dip you forefinger into a preparation of rosewater or Lavender essential oil. Give the water or oil a chance to warm on your fingertip.

Massage the oil gently into the third eye (the massage site of the pituitary gland), a point between and slightly above the eyebrows, making small clockwise circles to smooth the furrows from the brow.

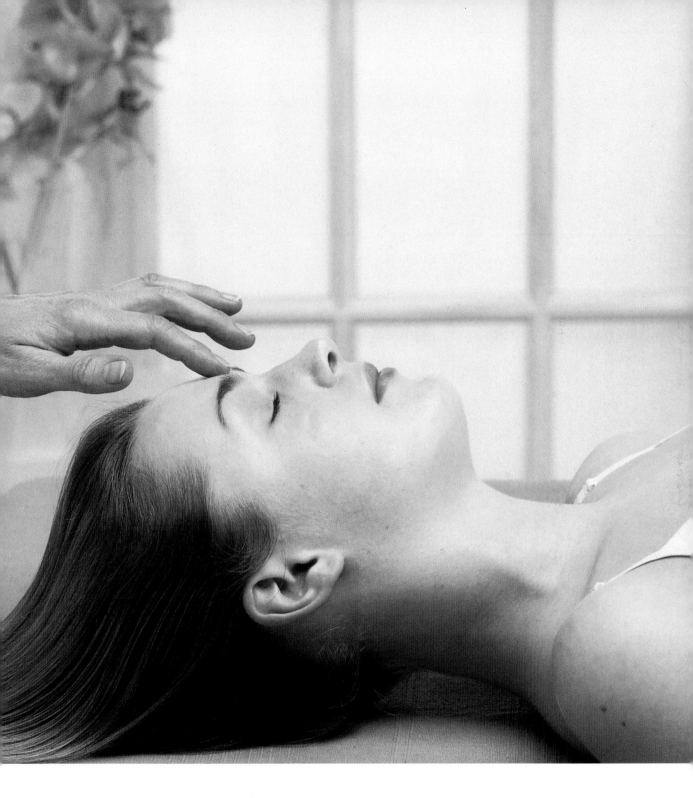

⌃ 28) closing the massage

As a finishing touch, gently press the third eye with your forefinger. Pause and release.

Variation *Cover the eyes and forehead with either a cold or warm cloth, sprinkled with scented oil or water.*

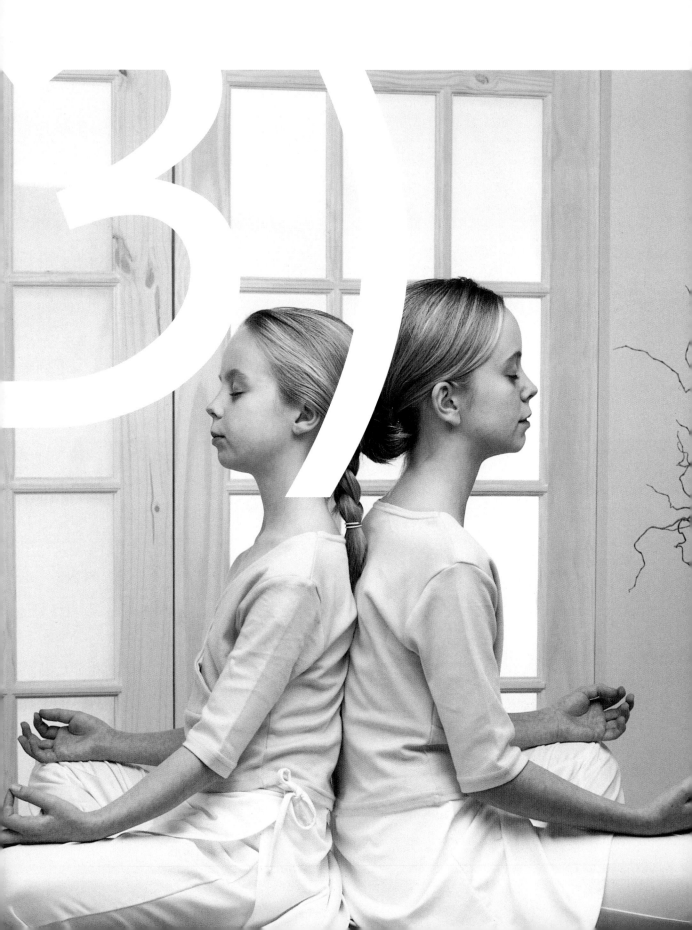

complete relaxation

3

complete relaxation

'The soul that moves in the senses, and yet keeps the senses in harmony, finds rest in quietness.'

Bhagavad Gita

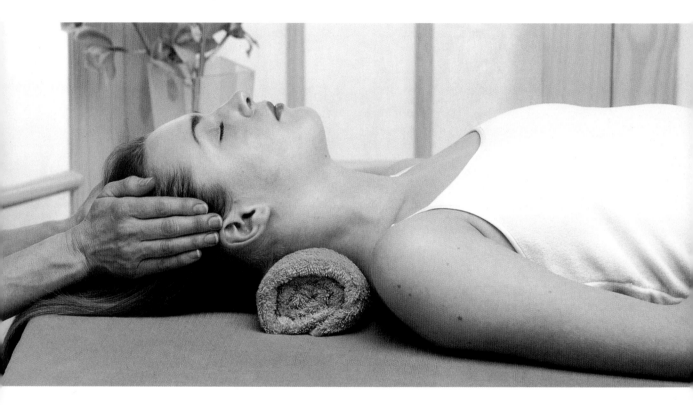

Our mental attitude and personal experiences are etched on our faces and mirrored in our eyes. Finding inner peace is a perfect way of staving off the ageing process as it softens the hard lines of living.

Going on a personal journey through the layers of your mind helps you to explore a whole inner world. Learning how to harness the powerful forces there with a compassionate heart in a relaxed body brings a state of complete relaxation. Without really trying, the specially arranged practices which follow will help you to tune in to the forces of gravity which allow Mother Nature to do her very best in absorbing any physical, mental or emotional pain.

physical detachment

1) Spine Sit on the floor or a large table. Roll back onto one elbow and then the other, relaxing vertebra by vertebra until the whole spine is lying flat. Extend and relax the lumbar region of the spine (lower back), feeling the pull of gravity.

2) Chest and lungs Open and expand your chest and lungs, especially the sternum area, the breastbone.

3) Head and neck Support your neck and head with a tightly rolled and folded towel (if your chin is not at right angles to your chest when you're lying down flat).

4) Throat Swallow to relax your throat, feeling the cool, incoming breath over the back of the throat, soothing the nerve endings to the brain.

5) Hands Rest the back of your left hand on your brow to help focus your thoughts while resting the other hand on a rolled towel. Once you feel sufficiently focused, rest the left hand on a towel.

6) Eyes Gently close your eyes, focusing your attention on the third eye.

7) Lips Lick and soften your lips, allowing them to part slightly. Relax your tongue from the roof of your mouth and ease your jaws apart.

8) Legs Rest the legs over a large round cushion or rolled blanket to help rest the lower back.

9) Whole body Surrender yourself to Nature's powerful healing forces.

mental detachment

Having started the journey with the first nine steps of bodily relaxation, we move on to mind adjustments – from tension into deep relaxation. Slowly, your relaxed body will encourage your mind to appreciate its real powers. Be patient: mind relaxation is a lifetime study and since peace of mind is ageless and timeless, trying to measure your attainment in terms of time is not appropriate. A truly relaxed mind flinches neither from life nor death. Through a quiet, informal but sincere attitude of mind, you can travel to the known and the unknown without any anxiety, living with security in insecurity.

Mentally say to yourself:

1) 'I detach my mind from my family ... I think of them lovingly then detach, relax and let myself go ... I detach my mind from those friends who take first place in my life ... I think of them lovingly ... detach ... relax ... and let myself go ... I detach my mind from my work and chores, I think of them ... detach ... relax and let them go.'

2) 'I hear no particular sound, as one sound blends beautifully into another ... I have no particular feelings ... no particular thoughts, as one thought is blending into another. Time itself is standing still for a split second of perfect stillness and perfect peace.'

Once this sense of timelessness is reached, it is equivalent to several hours' sleep. The results of your patient practice will be an air of calmness and deep serenity which will be invaluable in any therapy that you undertake.

tension in the eyes

Working to deadlines is a pressure which builds up and sometimes just won't go away. The end results are tension headaches, eyestrain and lack of mental focus which, if left unchecked, can greatly impair productivity. Taking a few minutes off every once in a while to do these self-help pressure-release techniques will prevent and relieve stress.

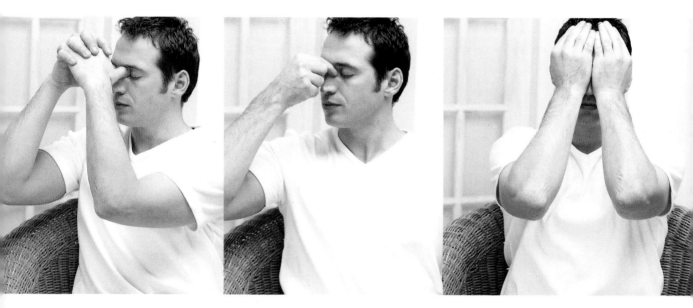

⌃ 1) pinching the eye socket

Lace your fingers and press your thumbs inside the corners of your eyes, just below the eyebrows. Hold for 2–3 seconds, release slightly and repeat six times.

Variation *Lean on your elbows to give more pressure to the action. Avoid any contact with the eyeball itself.*

benefit

Helps clear headaches and ease sinus problems.

⌃ 2) pinching the nasal bone

Pinch the top of the nasal bone (between the eyebrow and eye socket) with your forefinger and thumb. Hold the fleshy area for two or three breaths, release slightly and repeat six times.

Variation *Lie on the floor to allow gravity to absorb any discomfort while performing the pressure action.*

benefit

Opens and brightens the eyes, clears the vision, relieves tiredness.

⌃ 3) cupping

Rub your palms together until they feel really warm, then lightly cup over your eyes. Hold in place for a few breaths, feeling the flow of warming, healing energy. Repeat whenever you feel you need a boost.

benefit

Energizes the eyes and refocuses the mind.

tension in the neck

⌃ 1) occipital circling

Cradle the back of your head in your hands and circle your thumbs around the soft, fleshy area at the base of the skull. Work methodically around the area to your own level of comfort. Relax and repeat twice more after a short break.

benefit

Repeated application melts away tension in the neck.

⌃ 2) smoothing through the hair

Slide your fingers up from the base of the hairline at the back of the neck and over the crown. Gather your hair at the roots and tug gently from side to side, keeping your knuckles close to the scalp. If you have little or no hair, adapt the technique so that in the final position you move the scalp with strong pressure through the fingers.

Now slide your fingers through your hair from the temples to the sides of the head. Gather your hair and pull gently from side to side.

Repeat both steps two or three times. Finish by smoothing through the hair.

benefit

Lifts depression and mental frustration as well as drawing out the tension that builds up in the back of the neck.

dealing with headaches

The head is like a pressure cooker. As stress builds up, so does the pressure. Becoming hot and bothered exacerbates this natural process, as does grinding your teeth, squinting or even talking too much. All these habits contribute to headaches. The following sequence can help to relieve them.

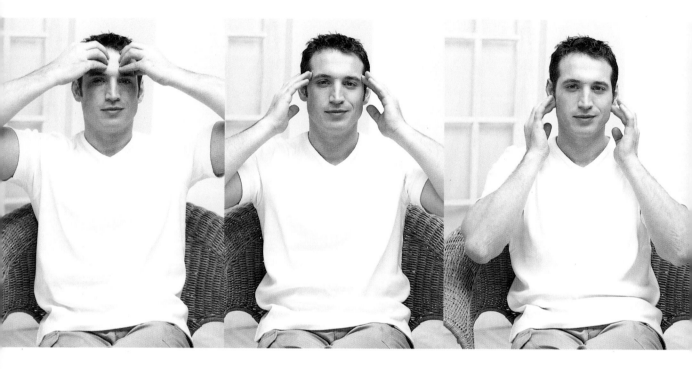

⌃ 1) pressing the forehead

Place the fingertips on your forehead, applying a little pressure. Stroke outwards from the centre to the temples. Repeat three times.

benefit

Smoothes away worry lines and eases emotional distress.

⌃ 2) circling the temples

Keeping your shoulders and elbows relaxed, place your middle fingers on the indentation of the temples. Gently massage them with small, circular movements six times.

benefit

Prevents and relieves headaches.

⌃ 3) releasing jaw tension

Still using the middle fingers, massage down the side of the face to the hinge of the jaw, just below the earlobes. Circle around the area. With someone who is particularly tense, keep going until you feel the jaw 'drop', and relax. Repeat six times.

benefit

Prevents and relieves the build-up of tension which causes neuralgia and headaches.

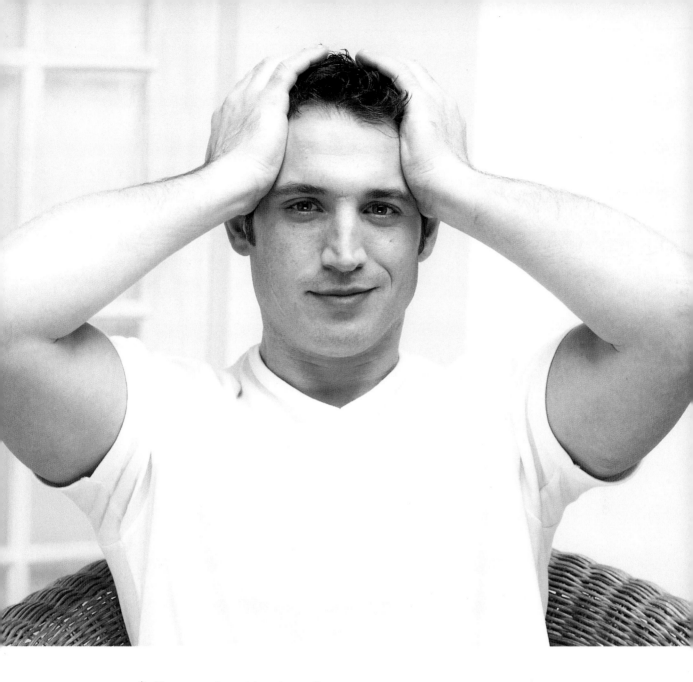

⌃ 4) pressing the temple

Fit the palms of your hands into the grooves of the temples. Squeeze gently with the heels of your hands and make slow, wide circles six times.

Variation *Take the circular movement over the cheekbones into the hollows of the cheeks and work into the face.*

benefit

Relieves and prevents headaches and facial tension.

relaxing at school

We don't always consider that our children need – or even can – relax. Like the rest of us, they suffer from the effects of timetables, homework and noisy environments. This series of steps is not only great fun for children, but also an effective way of learning how to relax and unwind. To do them, children need to work in pairs. The first three steps are designed to energize and uplift.

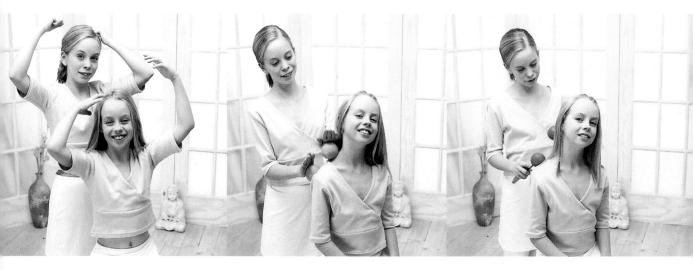

⌃ 1) wake-up call

Form soft fists with your hands and gently beat the head all over 10–15 times. Make sure to keep your wrists and hands very relaxed.

Variation *Beat the head lightly with your fingertips.*

benefit

Stimulates the supply of oxygen to the brain and makes you feel wide awake.

⌃ 2) smiley balls

Find two small, roundish oranges and roll them around the muscles of your partner's shoulders and back, applying firm pressure with your palms.

Variation *You could use tennis or soft rubber balls instead.*

Caution: Do not roll over the spinal vertebrae.

⌃ 3) extended balls

These rubber balls, available from some high street stores, are attached to flexible metal handles and can be used to break up the tight muscle areas of the back. Beat in a rhythmical way, alternating the balls, for a minute.

Variation *If you cannot obtain the extended balls, perform the alternate beating with two hand-held oranges or small, soft balls.*

benefit

Relieves deeper-seated tension in the back and shoulder muscles.

asthma, bronchitis and rounded shoulders

The percentage of children suffering from asthma and bronchitis is far too high, and increasing. Although triggered by pollution, smoky environments and genetic factors, the problem is nonetheless aggravated by uncorrected poor posture and inadequate desk and chair design. Working at a flat surface only encourages a 'caving-in' of the chest and a sinking into the hips. These stronger techniques help to give the body a safe natural traction and postural realignment.

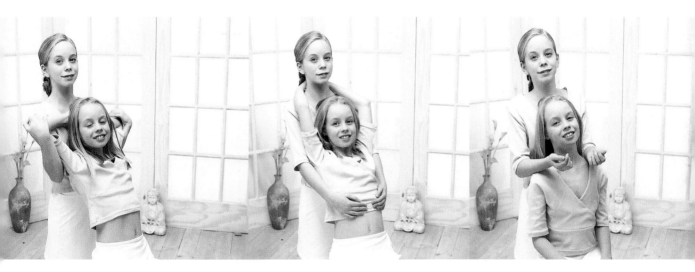

⌃ 4) expanding the chest

Sit your partner on a low stool with their hands clasped behind their head. Stand behind them to give support and cup their elbows in your hands. Simultaneously inhale and pull back the elbows, levering your body against your partner to help increase the stretch. Exhale, release slightly and repeat six times.

benefit

Prevents the tendency to rounded shoulders.

⌃ 5) stretching the body

Lace your partner's clasped hands behind your neck and cradle your hands around the lower part of their ribcage. Simultaneously inhale, leaning back to stretch and expand the torso. Exhale, release slightly and repeat six times.

benefit

Prevents the build-up of tension in the armpits and chest and energizes the whole body.

⌃ 6) pressing the shoulders

Press your forearms into your partner's shoulders. Hold for about 10 seconds, release slightly and repeat six times.

benefit

Helps to level the shoulders and ease neck and shoulder tension. This is one of the best antidotes to poor posture caused by children habitually carrying a bag on one favoured shoulder.

stiff and neglected joints and muscles

The early flexibility of youth is soon lost if the body is not used properly. Activities such as climbing trees and rolling down the hill are, for many, only a dream. The steps here act as a complete head-to-toe tonic and can soon help to revive and maintain a sense of suppleness. In the spirit of equality, encourage your partner to change roles with you after the completed series and receive the benefits in reverse.

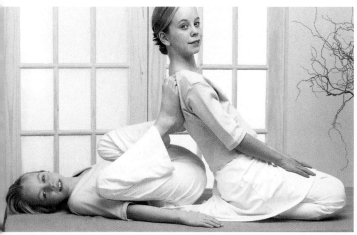

≪ 7) pressing the body

Ask your partner to lie flat on the floor, on their back, while you kneel close to their hips. Ask them to rest their feet on your ribcage, and then walk them up and down the muscles on either side of your spine, several times. Lean back into their feet, easing their knees open, and hold for two or three breaths. Release slightly and repeat three times.

benefit

Massages your back while easing your partner's hip, knee and ankle joints.

8) rise and shine ≫

With your partner still lying on their back, sit up against their buttocks. Their knees should be bent and slightly open, and their feet resting on your hips. With your hands on your thighs for support, invite your partner to walk their feet up the muscles on either side of your spine until their insteps are on your shoulders. As they walk their feet upwards, they should support the small of their back or the pelvic girdle with their hands (in this position, the upper arms and elbows form a framework which spreads the weight evenly). To relieve any pressure on the throat, they should make sure that their elbows are in line with their shoulders – and chin square to their chest.

benefit

Recharges the metabolism.

Caution: This exercise is not suitable for people with high blood pressure.

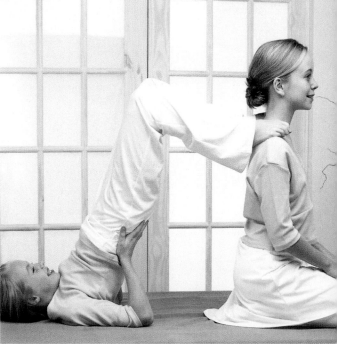

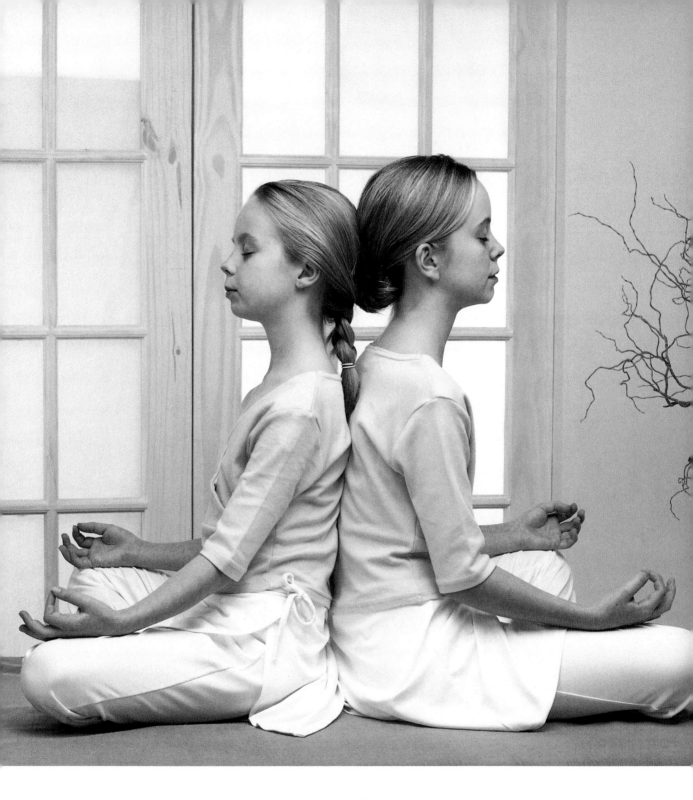

⌃9) resting and relaxing

Sit back-to-back with your bodies touching, legs folded in a cross-legged position. Sit on folded towels, if necessary, so that your knees are at a lower level than your hips. Close your eyes and tune into, and synchronize, your breathing patterns. Rest in the position, enjoying each other's warmth and support.

relaxing at home

So often we get home from work to be faced with yet more to do in the way of cooking and domestic chores – and in these circumstances, the last thing on our minds is how we can help ourselves to unwind. This easy bathroom routine can be fitted into the busiest schedule. All you need is a standard bath towel.

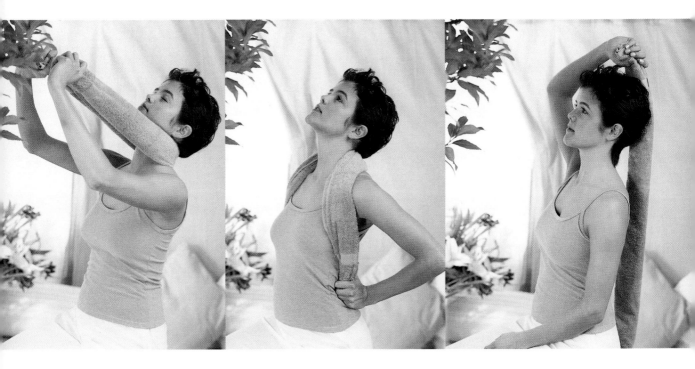

⌃1) stretching the neck

Cradle your neck in a warmed, rolled towel. Arch the head back and hold for two or three breaths.

⌃2) stretching the neck and shoulders

Pull the ends of the towel down and wrap it around your shoulders. Press your fists into the small of the back, pinching the elbows back to increase the pressure and expand the chest. Hold for two or three breaths. Repeat steps 1 and 2 six times.

benefit

Smooths and unravels the knots in the neck and shoulders.

⌃3) pressing the body

Sitting on the floor, hold the rolled towel down your spine. Tuck one end under your buttocks and hold the other end extended over your head. Slowly ease your body down onto the floor on top of the towel, centring your spine over the end. Release the top end of the towel, bend your knees and place your hands on your hips. Rest and relax, allowing the muscles on either side of the rolled towel to open and relax with the pull of gravity. Stay in this position for a few minutes. Any physical pain and tiredness can be dispelled in just a few minutes without doing anything.

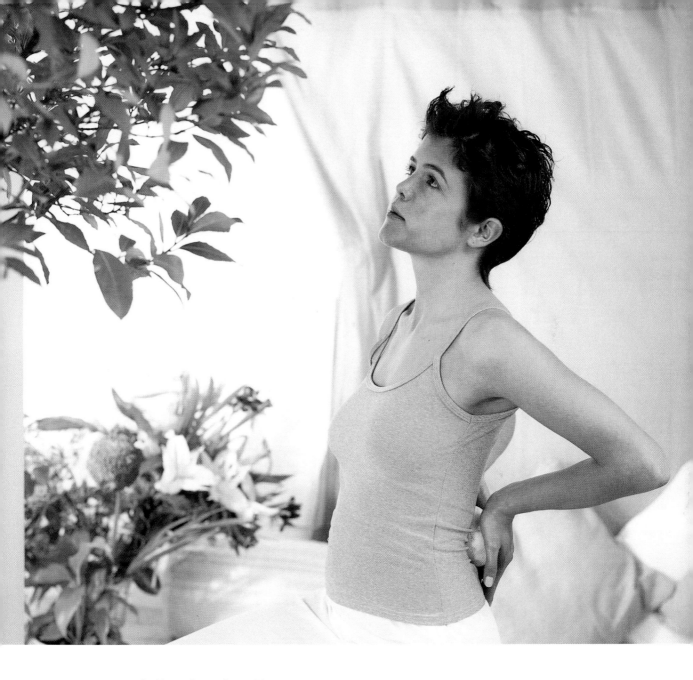

⌃ 4) releasing the pressure

Put two tennis or soft balls into a sock and knot the top.
  Press the balls into the tight muscles on either side of the spine and hold for two or three breaths.

Variation Use this technique to relieve the strain of long journeys by pressing into the back muscles while seated.
  Alternatively, lie on the floor with your knees bent, and tuck the balls under your back, against the.muscles on
  either side of the spine.

treating stiffness and injury

Unfortunately, a number of people are so constrained by chronic poor posture, pain, stiffness and injury that even lying on the floor or in a bed brings neither relief nor true relaxation. One of the best solutions I have found for treating such people is the on-site massage chair. In my opinion, it is the ideal choice for the professional masseur. Its design enables all-round access and your partner can instantly relax into the pull of gravity. Its surfaces support every part of the body while maintaining unrestricted posture.

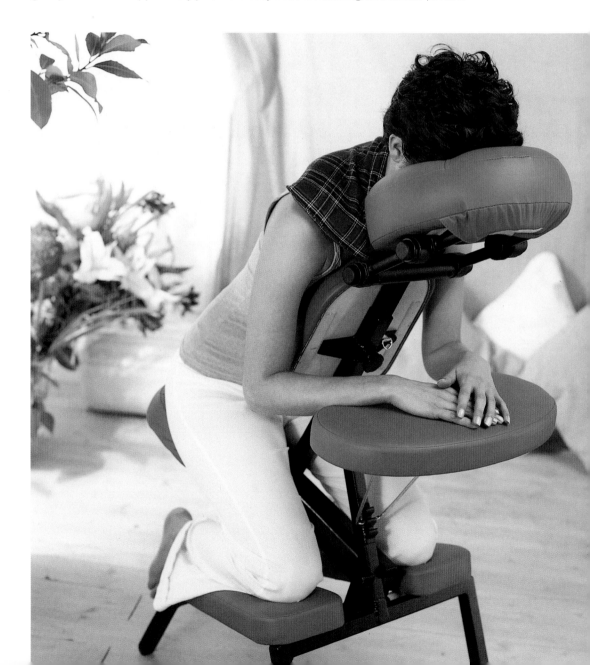

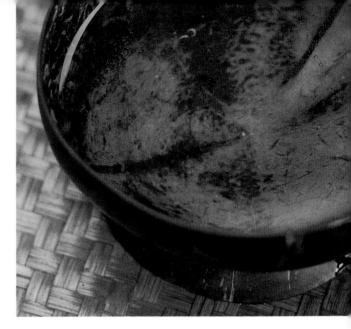

There will be occasions when your partner reports injury which would normally be a contra-indication against treatment. You are not entirely powerless in this situation and can provide a measure of relief quite safely in the form of a compress. These are an effective way of relieving pain, swelling and reducing inflammation. Generally hot compresses are used to treat chronic pain (backache and neckache, fibrocitis, rheumatic and arthritic pain, abscesses, earache and toothache) and cold compresses for acute pain (headaches, for example) and as a first-aid treatment for injuries and sprains (such as tennis elbow).

Of the recommended oils to treat muscular spasm, you may choose from the following selection, all of which are noted for their antispasmodic and relaxing qualities: Bergamot, Black Pepper, Camomile, Clary Sage, Fennel, Juniper, Lavender, Marjoram, Melissa, Neroli, Peppermint, Rosemary, Sandalwood and Thyme.

Of the recommended oils to treat muscular aches and pains, you may choose from the following selection, all of which are noted for their analgesic (pain-killing) effect and are essential muscle toners which can be applied prior to all strenuous sports and training, as well as being a relaxing tonic afterwards: Bergamot, Black Pepper, Camomile, Cinnamon, Eucalyptus, Lavender, Marjoram, Neroli, Pine, Rosemary and Sage.

Of the recommended oils to treat rheumatic aches, choose from the following: Bay, Camomile, Cedarwood, Eucalyptus, Juniper, Lavender, Lemon, Marjoram, Pine, Rosemary and Thyme.

To treat arthritis you may choose from the following selection, all of which are noted for easing painful inflammation of the joints, whether rheumatoid or osteoarthritic: Benzoin, Camomile, Cedarwood, Fennel, Juniper, Lavender, Lemon, Marjoram, Pine and Rosemary.

Preparing a compress

1) For a hot compress, fill a basin with 1.2 litres (2 pints) of water, as hot as your hands can bear. For a cold compress, use as cold water as possible, preferably cooled with ice.

2) If desired, add essential aromatherapy oils to the water. Use 4–5 drops for adults and 1–2 drops for sensitive skin.

3) Fold a piece of clean, absorbent fabric (lint, cheesecloth, unmedicated cotton wool, clean old sheeting or towelling) and soak it in the water, ensuring that surface oils (if used) are captured.

4) Wring out the excess water and place on the affected area.

5) When a hot compress has cooled to blood heat, remove it and replace with a new one. A cold one should be renewed when it has warmed to blood temperature.

releasing strain and increasing flexibility

⌃ 1) circling the head and neck

Warm your hands by rubbing them briskly together. Rest them lightly on your partner's shoulders. Centre yourself and pause as you connect and synchronize your breathing with that of your partner. Make wide circles around the shoulder muscles, gently breaking up any knotty areas. Repeat six times.

Make smaller circles as you progress up the neck muscles towards the base of the skull. Repeat six times.

⌃ 2) raking

Form a 'V' shape with the forefinger and middle finger of your working hand. Rest the mother hand comfortably on one shoulder. Starting at the base of the neck, press your fingertips with moderate pressure around the contours of the vertebrae, continuing down to the middle of the back. Finish by trailing the back of the fingers up either side of the spine. Repeat three times.

⌃ 3) flat-edge knuckling

Make soft knuckles with your fists. Gently knead, with the flat edge, across the shoulders and down the spinal muscles. Continue down the arms and repeat three times. Smooth over the area you have worked.

benefit
_____

Energizes the nervous system.

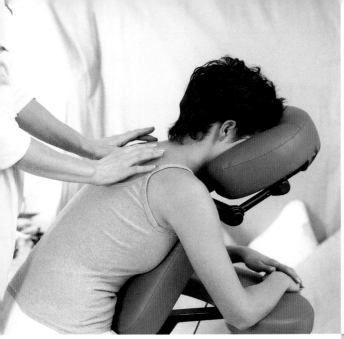

«4) feather stroking

Stroke down the neck, shoulders and spinal muscles with light, feather-like fingertips. Repeat two or three times.

5) smoothing up »

Using the backs of your hands, smooth up the back and neck, using long strokes. Repeat six times.

benefit

Leaves your partner feeling uplifted.

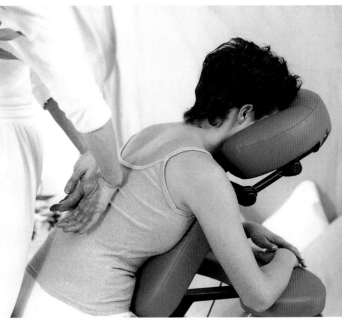

« 6) finishing touch

Leave your partner to rest for a few minutes. Cover them with a warm blanket or light cotton sheet for added comfort.

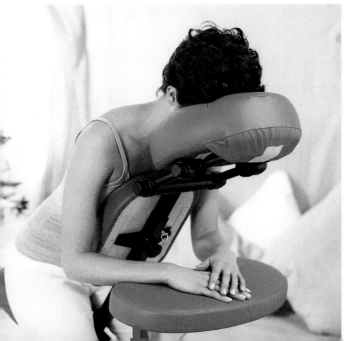

soothing and sensual

The prerequisite to all fulfilling and loving relationships is touch. It is that certain something that defines a real love affair. I find this aspect of communication with my partner a transforming and enriching one. No two people create the same vibration. The chemistry is always different. What does remain a constant is the willingness to give and take. These introductory tender touches might inspire you to an exploration of the sensual and erotic nature of any burgeoning or established relationship.

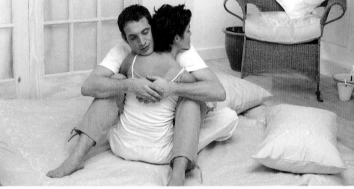

1) smoothing the back and neck »

Sit facing one another, interweaving your legs, and cradle one another's torsos in your arms. Overlap your hands and smooth around the back and neck in a clockwise or anticlockwise direction depending on your intuition or your partner's preference. Take it in turn, mirorring each other's movements and explorations.

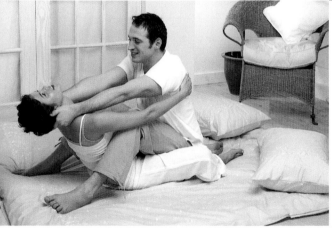

« 2) see-saw stretch

Support the back of your partner's neck with your hands. Their arms should be extended and secured in place behind your back. Ease your partner back as far as you can, then bring them upright. Repeat six times. Your partner then repeats the step in mirror fashion.

Now both clasp one another's necks as before, and lie back to the fullest extent you can manage. Rock backwards and forwards like a see-saw, taking your time and trusting yourself increasingly to your partner's support. Repeat as many times as you wish.

3) circling the temples »

Interlace your fingers around your partner's neck. Using gentle but persistent pressure, squeeze the heels of your hands into the muscles on either side of the neck. Hold for a few seconds, then release. Repeat several times, then allow your partner to perform the same step on you.

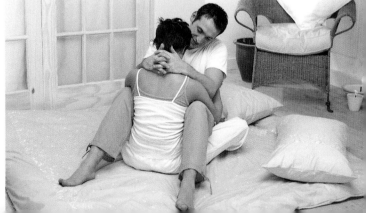

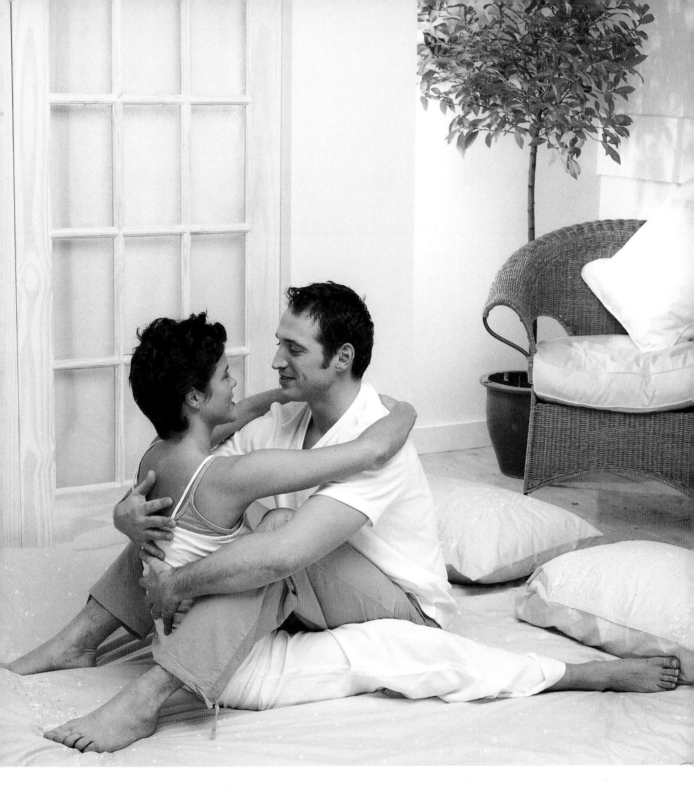

4) cuddling

Finish this series with a tender embrace, slowly gaining in intensity until your hearts and bodies are completely connected.

soothing and sensual

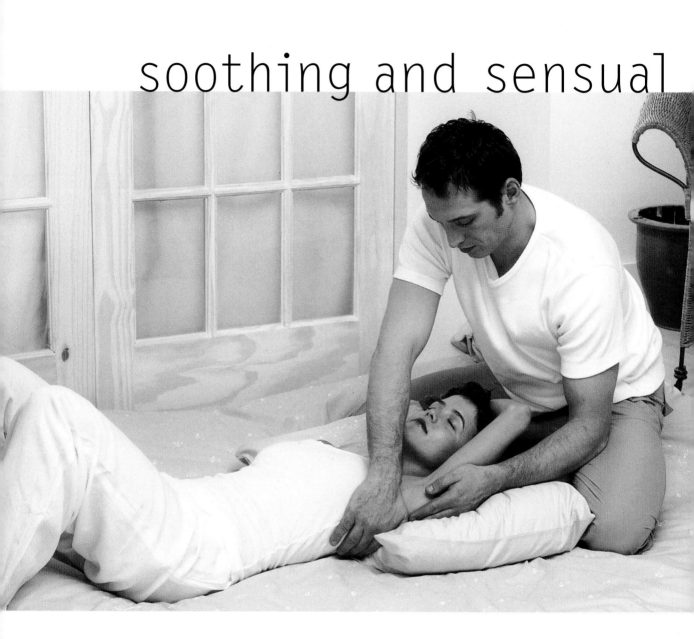

⩗ 5) smoothing through the arms

Ask your partner to lie on their back on the floor. Support the upper body and head with a cushion. Adopting an astride kneeling position as close to their head as possible, fold their left arm over the head. Slide your mother hand under the ribcage and place the working hand above it on the chest so that the chest is sandwiched between your two hands. Pulling both hands towards you, smooth up through the armpit and along the arm to the hand. Repeat two or three times. Repeat with the right arm.

benefits

Aids lymphatic drainage, as well as having a soothing and nurturing action.

6) smoothing and stretching through the arms »

Starting with both your partner's arms loosely folded over the head, slide both your hands under their ribcage. Pull slowly but firmly along the back of the ribs, through the armpits and along the upper arms. Continue the flow of the movement along the forearms and finish by gently grasping the wrists. Ensure that your hands enfold the back of the wrist rather than the pulse points. Lean back, stretching your partner's arms and shoulders, but only to their level of comfort – a gentle but persistent stretch would be appropriate. Release and repeat three times.

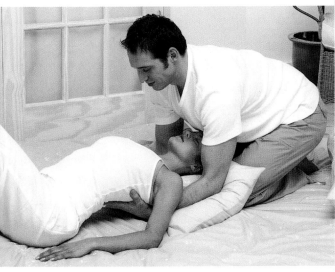

« 7) raking the upper back

Slide your hands under your partner's shoulder blades, spreading your fingers like flattened claws. Assist your partner to arch their back slightly as you rake your hands up the body and neck. Finish with a gently tailing off movement at the back of the head.

8) finishing touch: head and heart »

Very gently rest your working hand on your partner's heart and your mother hand on their forehead. Focus your attention on the interaction and energetic interplay between these two vital centres and your own.

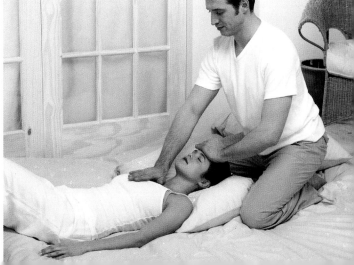

hi-ki natural face-lift

deep cleansing beauty routine

Beauty treatments do not have to be confined to a salon. You can have great fun experimenting with homemade preparations made from natural ingredients. Facial scrubs of ground nuts and lotions and masks of avocados or tropical fruit pulps all have enzymes which help to give the skin a whole new lustre. Working with self-prepared and freshly sourced organic products, rather than prepackaged ones, keeps you in touch with the vital forces of Mother Nature. Applying the potions with your fingertips or a natural bristle brush is an art in itself. Each stroke creates a rhythm and flow which massages the skin and soothes nerve endings, so that the recipient feels as if all their worry lines are being brushed away. The following deep cleansing beauty routine is one I use regularly. A selection of my recipes can be found on page 118.

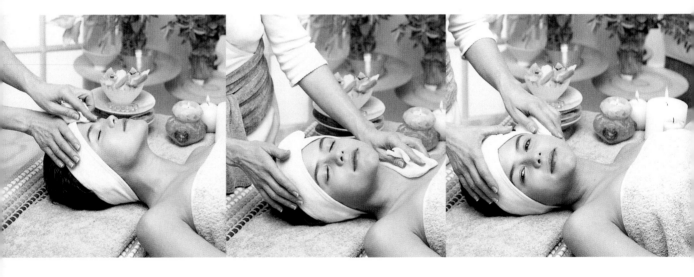

⌃ 1) cleansing the face

Prepare your partner by tying back their hair with a hair band or a head scarf. Cover the body with a warmed sheet and light blanket or a large bath towel. For comfort, you may also like to place a rolled or folded towel under the neck or head for support. Lightly soak a small piece of soft cotton cloth with some cleanser. Try two-thirds soya milk or coconut milk diluted with one-third of mineral water, filtered water or rain water. Gently work around the whole face with upward and circular movements.

⌃ 2) cleansing the neck

Ease your partner's head to one side and smooth upwards from the upper chest and over the side of the neck and face with the dampened cloth. Complete the sequence over the throat, chin, the side of the face and behind the ear. Repeat two or three times until this side of the face and neck are thoroughly cleansed, then turn the head and repeat the procedure on the opposite side.

⌃ 3) cleansing in and around the ears

Dampen a thin part of the cloth and work into the outer part of the ear with one finger, cleansing the tiny crevices with a light pressure. Finish with a complete circle around the base, in the crease near the skull. Cleanse both ears thoroughly in this way.

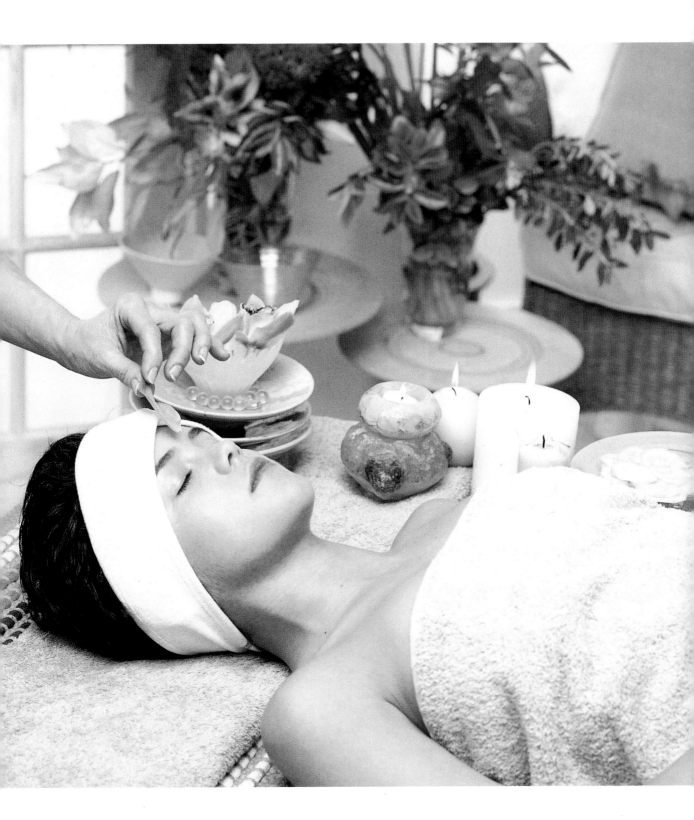

⌃4) soothing the face

Gently relax the facial muscles by smoothing over the contours with a scented rose petal or fine-textured flower.

deep cleansing beauty routine

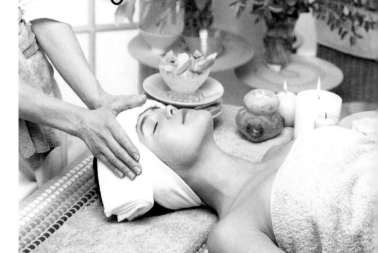

5) drying the forehead »

Arrange a folded pillowcase, made of plain or brushed cotton, into an oblong shape. Place over the forehead and sensitively smooth dry from the centre to the temples. Repeat two or three times.

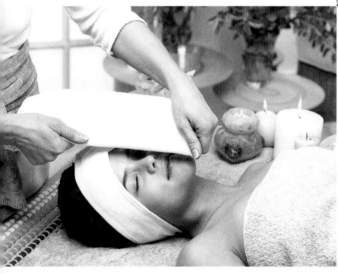

« 6) drying the side of the face

Place the short folded edge of the pillowcase down one side of the face, covering the nostril but not the nose, and bisecting the forehead. Lightly press your working forefinger down the contour of the forehead and the side of the nose. Then lightly smooth outward over the side of the face using the whole hand. Repeat on the other side of the face.

7) drying the neck and throat »

Place the folded pillowcase on the upper part of the chest. Hold the edge nearest to the neck and draw upwards over the surface of the throat and neck towards the chin. Repeat two or three times, drying the whole of the neck and throat. As a variation, make a tight roll and smooth over the throat with the same upward strokes.

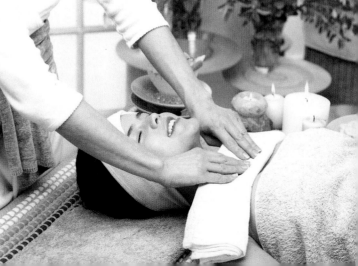

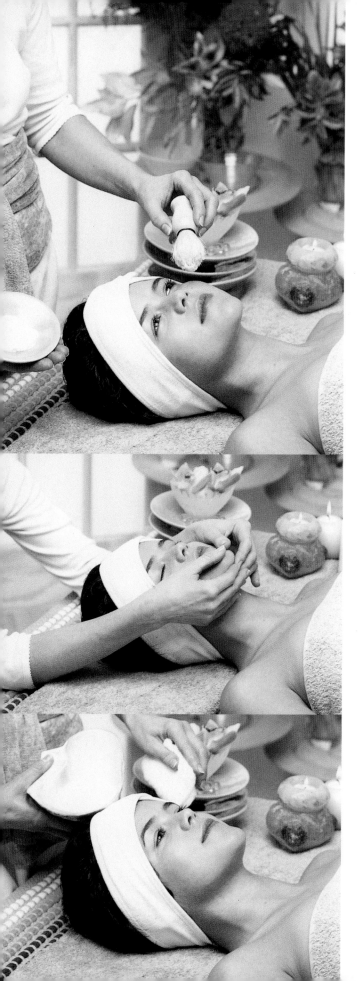

« 8) applying a scrub

Using medium pressure on the face and lighter pressure around the neck, apply your favoured pre-prepared scrub with a natural bristle shaving brush, avoiding the orbits of the eyes and the lips

« 9) massaging in the scrub

Work the scrub into the neck and throat with light, upward finger strokes. Work the chin with a light massage, using small circular movements. Continue with the circular movements until you have covered the whole of the face, again avoiding the orbits of the eyes and lips.

benefit

The scrub removes and breaks up dead skin and stimulates the natural secretion of oils. This helps to prevent drying and ageing of the skin. Even oily skin needs exfoliating. For this type of skin, use a lighter lotion with a touch of fresh lemon or lime juice.

« 10) washing off the scrub

Wash off the scrub with a small, rough flannel, wrung out in warm or cold rain water or mineral water. Alternatively use the 'milk' from two tablespoons of oatmeal soaked in 600 ml (1 pint) of hot water and strained. Gently dry the face with a warmed hand towel, lightly scented with rosewater.

deep cleansing
beauty routine

I very often apply progressive facial masks in the same session – some to deeply cleanse and dry, others to enrich and nourish. One of the rationales behind this concept is the removal of the 'metaphysical' masks that we all use to project a false or incomplete image to the world. Such behaviour can become habitual, leaving many afraid to show their natural beauty. This simple process can help you to rediscover your natural beauty – a soft, shining face with fresh vigour. Make your choice from one of the mask formulas on page 118.

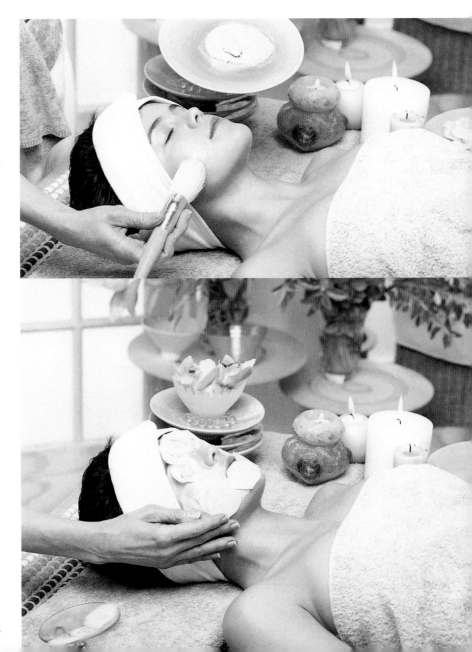

11) applying a facial mask »

Using a softer natural bristle make-up brush, make gentle circular movements over the face as you apply the preparation. Avoid the orbits of the eyes and the lips.

12) setting the mask »

To keep the mask moist once applied, cover the face with thin slices of peeled cucumber. Leave the mask to rest for about 10 minutes.

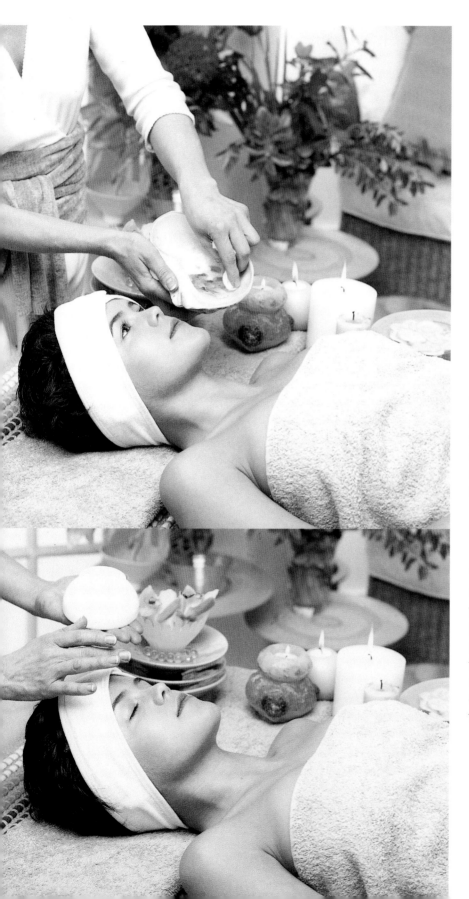

« 13) removing the mask

Remove the sliced cucumber and the surface mask preparation with a cloth dampened with filtered warm or cold rain water, mineral water or rosewater. Pat the face dry with a warm, soft hand towel.

« 14) nourishing and nurturing

Warm some rich face cream by using the back of your hand as a palette, or warm it in a small ceramic bowl over hot water. Apply the cream with your middle fingers, starting at the forehead. Circle outwards, moving down to the temples and then gently around the eye sockets and closed eyelids.

deep cleansing beauty routine

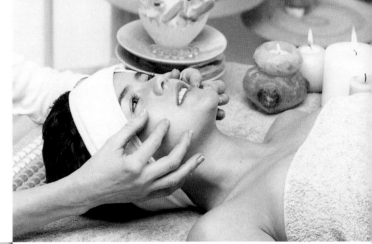

15) lifting the cheeks »

Moisten your fingertips with more warmed face cream and smooth across the cheeks in circular strokes, working from the nose outwards. Lift and release the cheek muscles, starting near the nostrils and moving out to the temples.

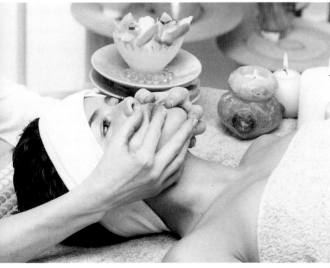

« 16) smoothing the lips

Replenish your fingers with more cream, if necessary. Gently press your thumbs onto the upper lip under the nose, and your forefingers under the lower lip. Cradle the jaw with your palms and relax the other fingers naturally under the chin. Smooth your fingers and thumbs outwards and upwards towards the temples. Circle the hollows of the temples with your index fingers. Gently press, pause and release. Repeat the whole process three times.

17) smoothing the chin »

Gently pinch the fleshy part of the chin between your thumbs and forefingers. Smooth and ease along the jaw to the temples, finishing with a circle. Press, pause and release. Repeat three times.

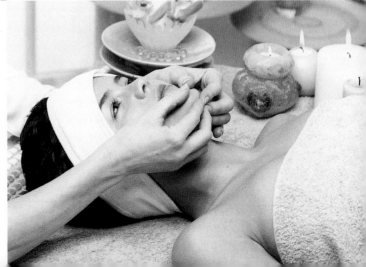

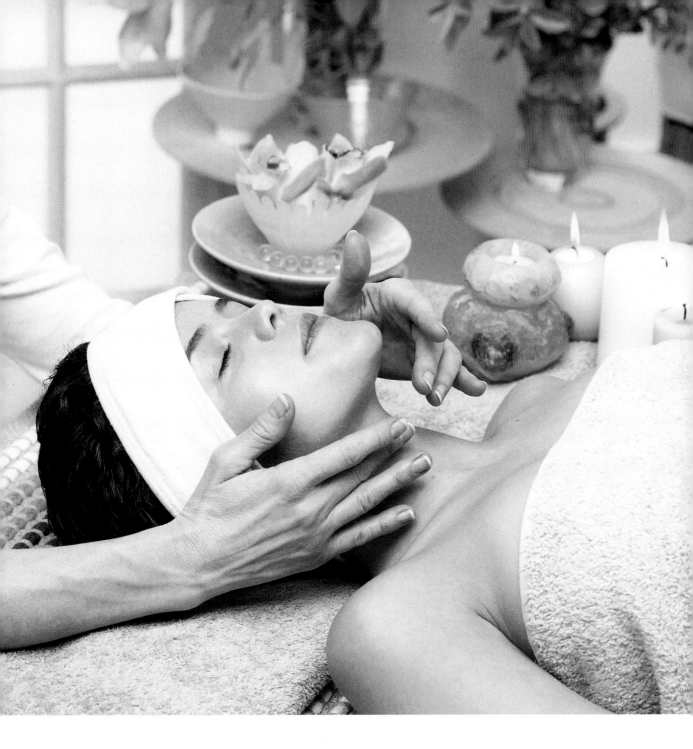

⊼ 18) smoothing the neck

Massage cream into the throat and neck with your fingertips, using light, upward strokes and alternating your hands. As a finishing touch, moisten an index finger and run it up from the tip of the nose to the third eye. Circle and press gently, pause and release.

Joseph Corvo's
10-minute massage

Every student of body work will know – or learn – that the physical structure of the body is but one aspect of a human being. Every ancient medical and healing system acknowledges an additional 'ethereal' dimension – that energetic component that complements and reflects the physical and is known as *ki, chi* or *prana*. As scriptural tenets and the ever-refreshed daily testimony of practitioners reliably inform us, this most intimate energy is the sustenance of our whole being. With knowledge and by improving practice, *ki* may be manipulated, directed and redirected to clear blockages and pave the way for expanded awareness and physical beauty. Its unimpeded, natural flow is essential to physical, emotional and mental wellbeing.

Balancing the vital energies

If the delivery of this energy is out of balance, nerve endings can become blocked and choked. Not enough blood, oxygen, protein and minerals reach the face, leading to dry, flaccid and ageing skin. Joseph Corvo's 'zone therapy' approach, which he developed into a daily 10-minute facial massage, can correct these imbalances, leading to improved muscle-building and more vital skin tone.

Since we are largely judged by our most visible feature – the face – its rigorous maintenance is probably the most rewarding beauty routine. Creams, lotions, cleansers and other skin-health products can only help so much. Manipulation is by far the most effective toner. If you want your face to be firmer, fuller, more handsome or beautiful, take the time to include this routine in your daily care regime. Your face will love you for it.

Locating the precise points

The zones of the body might vary slightly between individuals; however, if you perform these techniques regularly you'll soon intuit the exact locations. If you can't quite place the exact spot, go slightly above or below or to the side. In the initial stages you will soon discover the exact spot because it is likely to be sore or sensitive due to accumulated toxins. Make sure your nails are reasonable short so you do not lacerate your skin.

Applying pressure with sensitivity

Always massage with an upward and outward circular movement. You can work quite deeply on the points with a very firm action, according to your personal tolerance – some people can take more pressure than others. For all points apart from 3, 4 and 15, for which you must use a more gentle massaging movement, you can press as hard as you like without feeling uncomfortable. Where there is a lot of congestion, you will have to be sensible. Do not apply consistent pressure for long periods over hurtful spots. Give a few seconds' pressure, move on and come back to the tender place after a short rest. As your therapy progresses you will eliminate crystalline deposits from the skin and nerve endings until there is no further tenderness. Then you will know that the Zone Therapy approach has indeed worked.

Before you start the treatment, wash or cleanse your face and dry thoroughly. The pictures opposite indicate where you should massage and in what order. Spend about 30 seconds on each point.

Right: The pressure points on the face and ears. The numbers relate to the steps on the following pages.

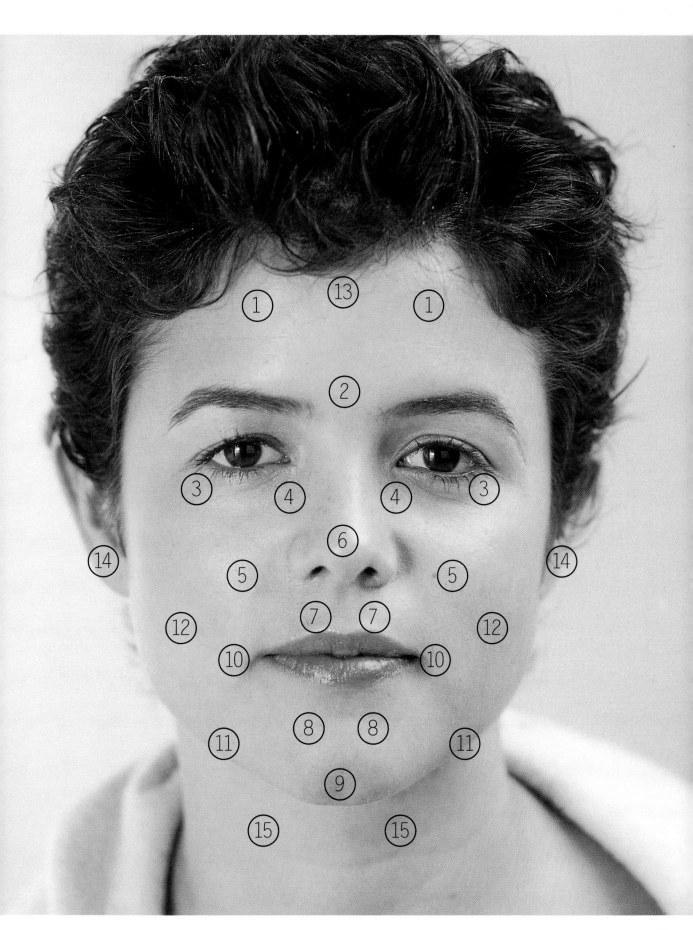

Joseph Corvo's
10-minute massage

⋀ 1) mental stimulation

This first position improves the skin and muscle tone of your forehead and improves mental awareness. Stress and worry lines etched into the forehead can, in time, be eliminated to no more than ghost-marks indicating previously fixed patterns of expression. Massaging this area, it is also believed, can improve your thinking processes and activate your reflexes.

technique

Find the upper edge of the forehead, where the bone indents. Then, starting at the sides, move slowly in towards the centre of the forehead, using your middle fingers and working in firm upward and outward circles of about 1 cm (½ in) wide. When you reach the centre, move outwards again. Complete four times.

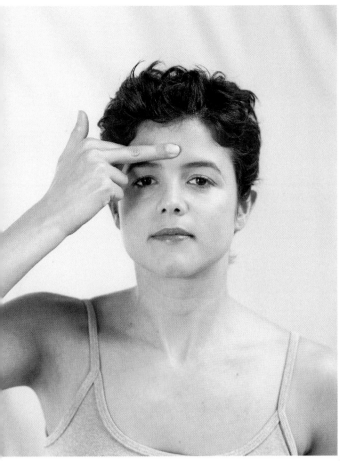

≪ 2) the pituitary gland and third eye

The pituitary gland is the crucial control centre which regulates the flow of hormones in the body. Traditionally associated with the master *Ajna chakra* – the third eye – its correct functioning is vital to the proper regulation of the whole endocrine system. Applying pressure here not only stimulates the pituitary gland but can also enliven your imagination and greatly improve your perception.

technique

Find the slight indent in your forehead. Massage in a small circle, about 1 cm (½ in) across for thirty seconds.

3) the colon ≫

Look after your colon and it will look after you. When it malfunctions, toxins will build up internally because waste matter is not being eliminated properly. Sluggishness and tiredness will result and the face will reflect this.

technique

To massage the pressure point 3, tap gently underneath each eye, starting on the outside and moving inwards towards the nose, then out again. Complete four times.

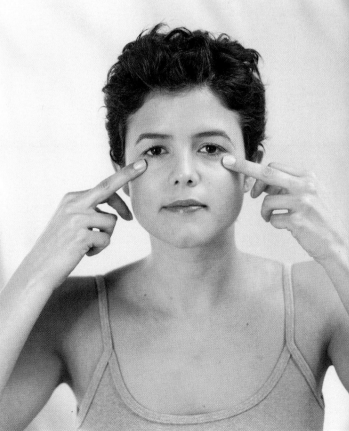

Joseph Corvo's 10-minute massage

4a) kidney stimulation »

Healthy kidneys eliminate toxins and acidity. Since most of the food we eat has a good deal of acidity, it is easy to see how vital these organs are. Any abnormality will affect a person's general health and the skin on the face will suffer very badly. Pressure point 4, beneath each eye, is linked to the kidneys.

technique

To massage pressure point 4, tap gently underneath each eye, starting on the outside and moving inwards towards the creases between the corners of the eyes and the nose, then out again. Complete four times.

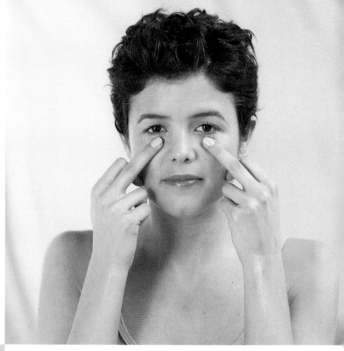

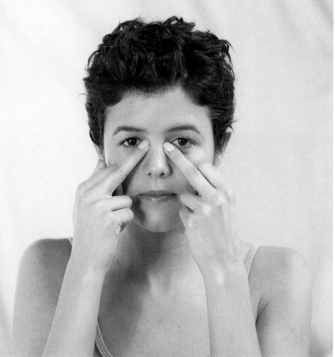

« 4b) kidney stimulation

technique

To massage pressure point 4, tap gently underneath the eye, starting on the outside and moving inwards towards the creases between the corners of the eyes and the nose, then out again. Complete four times. The picture illustrates the final position.

5) healthy bowel action »

Sluggish bowels are one of the main reasons for dull-looking, pasty skin. A thorough massage of the appropriate pressure points will stimulate and regulate bowel function, leading to glowing skin.

technique

Find the ridge of the cheekbone at its highest point, then press up into it. Massage as hard as you can in an upward and outward circular movement, while moving slowly along the length of the cheekbone. Complete four times.

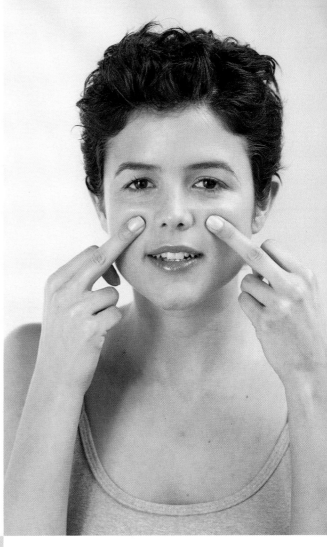

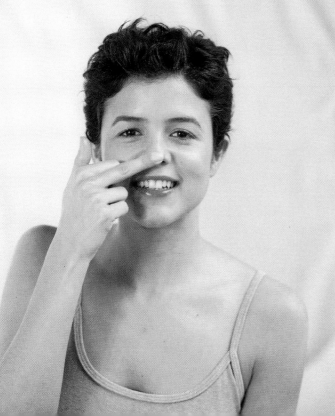

« 6) stomach problems

This step can be a great help to anyone suffering digestive troubles. A vigorous massaging of the nose tip will work wonders. Again, it is about unblocking those nerve endings.

technique

From step 5 and without lifting the finger of one hand, slide it up to the nose tip. Within the bounds of reasonable comfort, press as hard as you can and rotate slowly for 30 seconds.

Joseph Corvo's
10-minute massage

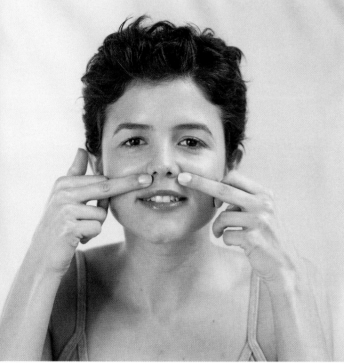

≪ 7) the spleen

One of the primary functions of the spleen is to remove worn-out blood cells. A healthy spleen is a prerequisite to maintaining a healthy stomach, so be sure to massage these areas thoroughly.

technique

Pressing inwards on either side of the ridge that runs from your nose to the middle of your upper lip, rotate your fingers in 1 cm (½ in) circles. Press hard so that you feel your gums beneath your fingers. Complete four times.

8) the pancreas ≫

The pancreas secretes alkaline enzymes which help the digestive process. A malfunction can cause too much acidity which is extremely harmful to the skin. Massaging these areas thoroughly can help you to attain and maintain a beautiful skin and face.

technique

Starting at the outer corners of the underside of the lower lip, work inwards with a firm rotating motion towards the centre, then out again. Press firmly enough to feel your gums beneath your fingers. Complete four times.

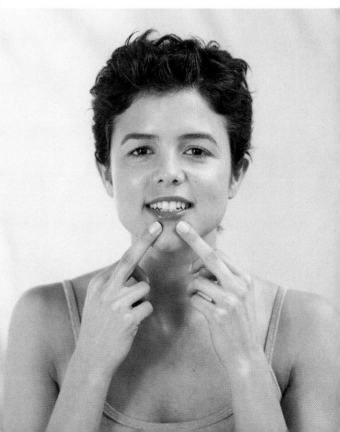

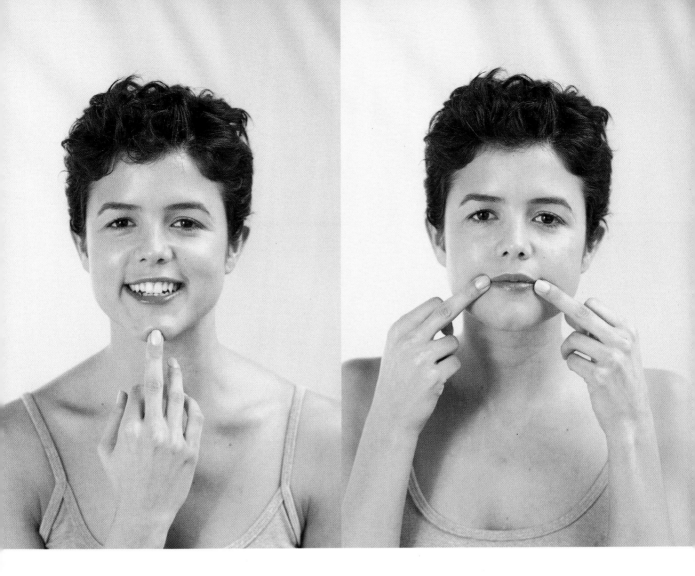

《 9) the bowels

Those who suffer from constipation are well aware of its pernicious effects on the body. It is one of the main causes of sluggishness and lack of energy. It also leads to a build-up of large amounts of toxins which results in lacklustre skin and eyes and unpleasant breath. Vigorous massaging of this area will greatly help to rectify the condition and bring back life and colour to the face.

technique

Find the indent in your chin, then rotate as firmly as you can bear for 30 seconds.

《 10) the lungs

Massaging the area associated with the lungs will ensure more efficient functioning of these organs and will help to ward off infections such as colds and debilitating conditions such as bronchitis and asthma which are often caused by stress. An improved supply of oxygen will greatly improve facial tissue quality and result in a more energized body generally.

technique

Find the muscle running down the length of the side of the mouth. Then, using a rotating motion, press inwards and outwards as hard as you can bear for 30 seconds.

Joseph Corvo's
10-minute massage

⌃ 11a) sexual desire

The healthy functioning of our sexual glands is indispensable to physical, emotional and psychological health. Their failure can lead to impotence, lack of sex drive and lack of control. When these glands (ovaries and testes) are functioning properly, it brings a glow to face and skin.

technique

Starting immediately below the ears, rub with a rotating movement along the ridge of the jawbone until you are directly underneath the pupils of the eyes. Work back again and repeat four times, pressing as hard as you can. The picture illustrates the starting position.

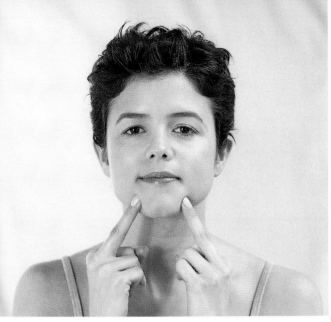

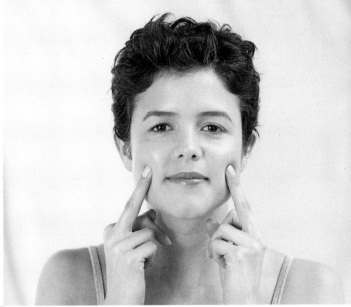

≪ 11b) sexual desire

technique

Starting immediately below the ears, rub with a rotating movement along the ridge of the jawbone until you are directly underneath the pupils of the eyes. Work back again and repeat four times, pressing as hard as you can. The picture illustrates the final position.

12) the liver and lymphatic system ≫

The liver helps to purify the blood. A sluggish liver affects the entire body, especially the facial skin. Sagging skin and a face that looks older than it should is the result of lack of proper nourishment. These movements also tone up the lymphatic system which is important to general health as well as to a lovely face and skin.

technique

Find the deepest pit of the cheek, where the jawbone meets the cheekbones. Massage in 1 cm (½ in) circles, pressing as hard as you can, for 30 seconds.

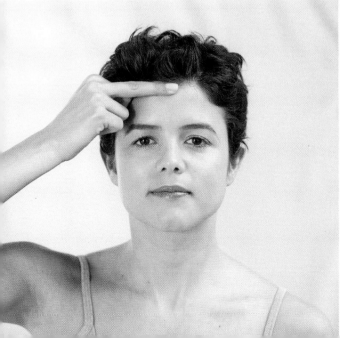

≪ 13) the sympathetic nervous system

Massaging this area tones up the whole nervous system and brings a sense of peace and tranquillity. This feeling of wellbeing is always reflected in the face.

technique

Massage the centre point on your forehead, working in 1 cm (½ in) circles and pressing as hard as you can, for 30 seconds.

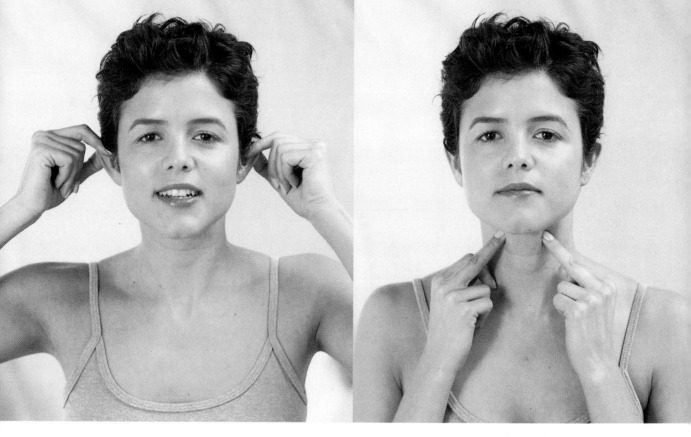

⌃ 14) toning up the entire body

Finally, tone the entire body by working on the ears. Like the feet, they contain many meridian node points relating to various parts of the body and its functioning.

technique

Massage both ears in turn by taking the entire ear between fingers and thumb. Start at the top and work up and down four times, pressing as hard as you can. After a few minutes your whole system will be pervaded by a glowing tingle. The effect will be seen in the facial muscles and the general tone of the face. The picture illustrates the final position.

⌃ 15) the thyroid

The thyroid points are situated on either side of the windpipe. They are vital to good health for, if they fail to work properly, the body becomes sluggish, the heartbeat is lowered and breathing becomes laboured. Sufferers feel the cold intensely and may put on weight; their circulation is poor and their skin becomes dry and scaly. They may also be distressed and unhappy and suffer several other unwanted symptoms including poor memory and problems with menstruation.

technique

To avoid all these ills and enjoy beautiful skin, work gently but well over the thyroid gland points. Starting on either side of the thyroid points, move inwards and upwards with a gentle circular movement. Complete four times.

Finishing touches

It is important that, after each 10-minute session, you drink a glass of water. This will help flush out the toxins you have dislodged in the skin and facial tissues.

If you follow Joseph Corvo's 10-minute facial massage and take the time to include it in your daily beauty routine, you will be assured of a stunningly more vital appearance. Massaging the pressure points regularly will give your face an entirely new and emollient look. Your muscle tissue and skin will firm up and give you a truly natural face-lift. True beauty comes from within and, after this routine, even a plainer-featured person will find that they exude an attractive energy which entices sexual partners, inspires confidence in others, accurately mirrors their emotions and correctly conveys their thoughts.

Although the sequence of pressure points are activated on the head, the effects are really system-wide. For instance, if you are overweight you should notice a slimming effect around hips, thighs and stomach. Reflexology, the foot-massage therapy, is gaining many converts for its evident success in regulating and treating the body's systems. The head, like the feet, is rich in accessible meridians and *chakra* energy nodes. Using a mirror for the initial orientation of your fingers, it is extremely simple to locate and freely massage these vital areas.

Positive affirmation

As with all systems that work on both a physical and mental level, establishing your expectations and the gentle discipline you need to perform this massage regularly are best accomplished with a positive affirmation. This should be kept brief and to the point and should use only positive and aspirational words. I offer here a couple of phrases my students have used so effectively over the years: 'My face is a picture of health and beauty,' and 'My skin is glowing with an inner radiance.'

Positive affirmations or Yogic/Tantric *Sankalpas* (great thoughts) harness the force of the mind, whose suggestive power is credited with all manner of self-cures and self-improvements. Where your mind leads your body will follow. If you visualize your skin as a perfect and vital organ you will be encouraged to put in the small increment of time required to achieve this state. I never cease to be amazed at how people can change their health and lifestyles around simply by the power of thought. Joseph Corvo has devised a natural face-lift sequence I can heartily recommend.

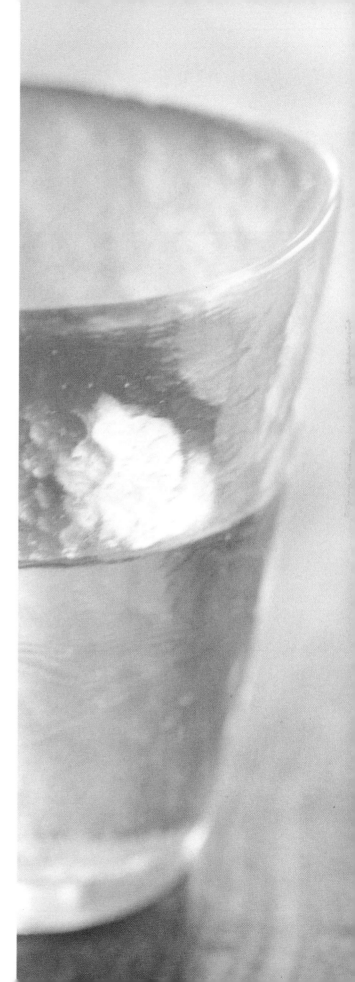

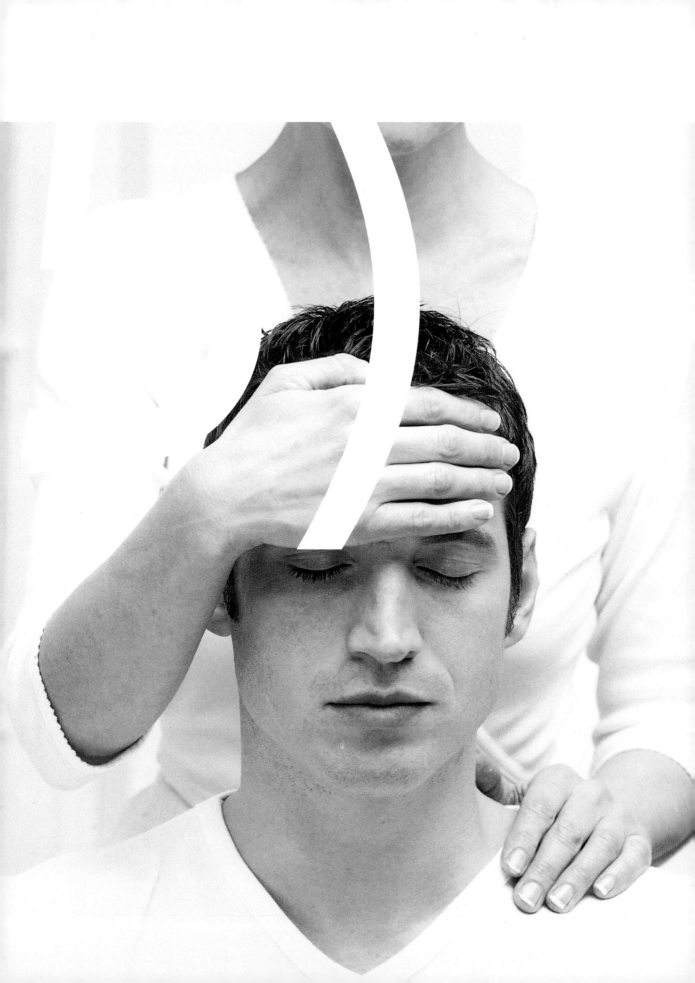

the healing power
of massage

(5

head wrapping routine 1

Enfolding the head in a scented pillow has an almost hypnotic effect. The sound of hands working against fabric helps to soothe and calm the nerve endings. I usually only use cotton or fine linen. Severe tension headaches, depression and anxiety can all be alleviated and prevented with this routine. The added bonus is that the treatment is less invasive to a sick person than direct hand massage, which they may find too much to cope with initially.

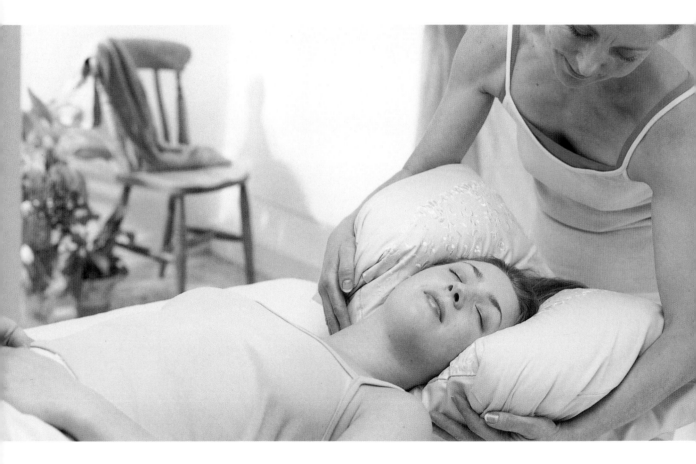

⌃1) pillow talk

If you want to continue this treatment into routines 2 and 3, prepare by laying an oblong piece of voile or fine cloth, as long as your extended arms, across the top of the bed or massage couch. Lay a single cotton sheet over this, rolled up widthways. Place a pillow on top. All the fabrics can be lightly scented with rose, lavender or orange flower water.

Ask your partner to rest their head on the pillow, with the hair away from the back of the neck. Slide your hands under the pillow and cradle their head, pressing inwards against the sides of the face. Hold for two or three breaths.

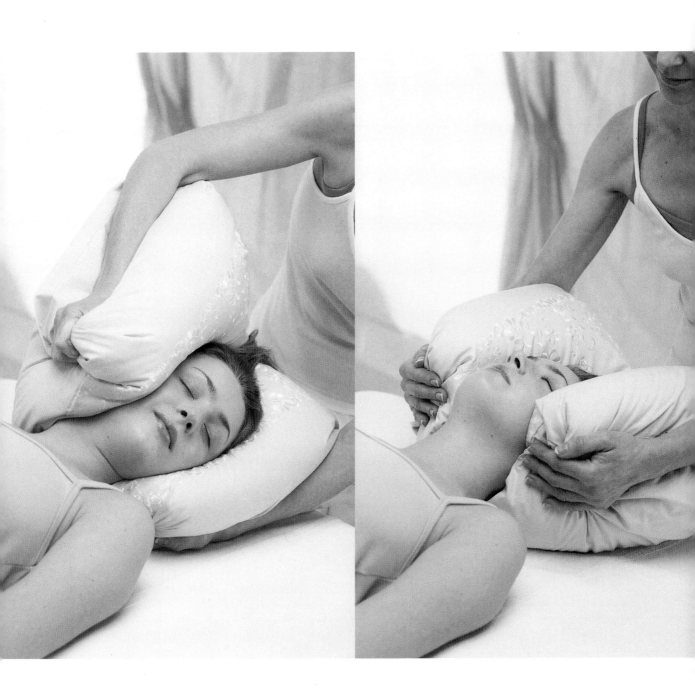

⌃ 2) twisting and turning

Using the pillow as support, turn the head to the right, then back to
the centre and over to the left. Repeat two or three times to help ease
the neck.

Caution: Keep the crown in line with the spine, especially in the turning movement.

⌃ 3) pulling off

Centralize the head and slowly pull the pillow away from under it,
tightening slightly on the back of the neck as you do so. If it is not already
there, place the roll of cotton sheeting under the neck for the next treatment.

head wrapping routine 2

1) pulling the head »

Slowly and gently pull the rolled sheet back towards you. Stretch the back of the neck and encase the ears and side of the head. Hold the stretch for two or three breaths, giving your partner time to relax and let go.

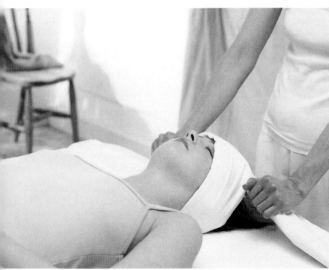

« 2) crossovers

Still holding the rolled sheet, cross your hands to fold the sheet over the forehead. Slide your hands under the base of the skull and smooth up over the fabric, gently pressing the ears and temples in a long stroke. Repeat two or three times. Unravel the fold and pull the rolled sheet away from under the head, holding it close to the sides of the head.

3) pressing the head »

Arrange the sheet over the top of the head, around the face, into the shoulders and along the arms. Press your palms into the top of the head and slide them down along the fabric, over the sides of the face towards the shoulders. Repeat three times.

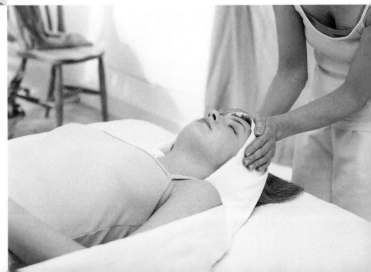

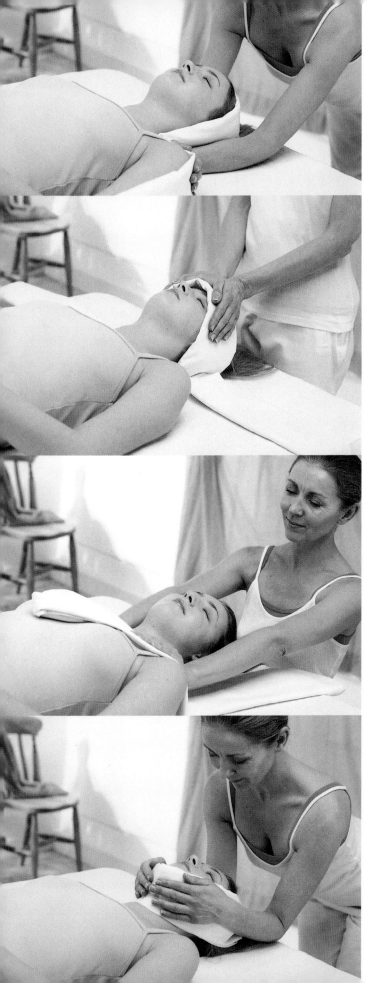

≪ 4) pushing the shoulders

Press your palms into the shoulders, easing down in the direction of your partner's feet. Hold for two or three breaths, slightly release and repeat three times.

≪ 5) pressing the forehead

Lift the rolled sheet and place over the brow, tucking it in around the temples and smoothing it off across the bed. Place your palms on the forehead and smooth outwards from the centre with both hands, moving over the temples to the sides of the head. Squeeze gently. Hold for 2–3 seconds. Repeat three times, ending the last movement by stroking out along the rolled sheet to the edge of the bed.

≪ 6) pushing the shoulder muscles

Pull the centre of the sheet, near the chin, down onto the centre of the breastbone, smoothing the roll over either shoulder. Push the shoulder muscles down towards your partner's feet. Release slightly and repeat three times.

To finish, lift the centre of the sheet upwards, pulling it lightly over the face and stroking either side of the face with the fabric.

≪ 7) smoothing the chin and jaw

Encase the chin and sides of the face with the rolled sheet. Cradle your hands around the chin and jaw. Smooth up over the fabric to the temples and press slightly. Hold for a few seconds and repeat three times.

head wrapping routine 3

These head-wrapping routines can be practised with different coloured cloths lightly perfumed with a variety of scented waters. Although there can be no hard-and-fast rules for colour therapy because each meridian may require a particular quality for balance, in general a colour's action either calms (pink), cools (blue), stimulates and energizes (red/orange), mentally refreshes and stimulates (yellow), invigorates (soft to vibrant greens), heals (lavender/violet), or purifies (white).

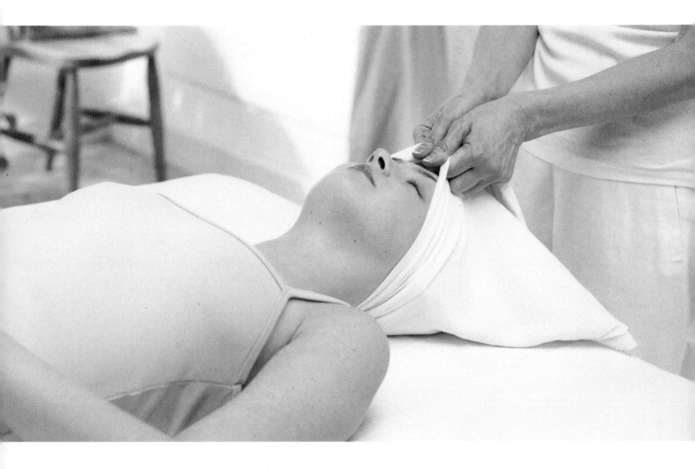

⋀ 1) pulling the head

Using the oblong piece of cloth placed beneath the head earlier, pull it back to encase the base of the skull and stretch the head and neck. Hold for two or three breaths, release slightly and repeat three times.

Variation: Grasp the sides of the cloth a hand's length back from the head. It still applies pressure but means you are not so close to the head.

2) knotting >>

Wrap the cloth over the head and twist, slightly pulling the hair; knot the cloth into the hair if it is long enough. Stand close to the knot to hold it in place with your body. Slide your hands down under the back of the skull and smooth up over the ears and temples. Repeat three times.

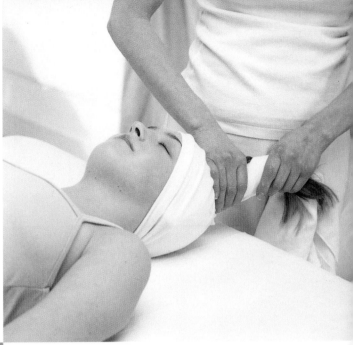

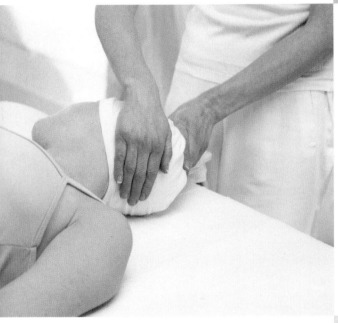

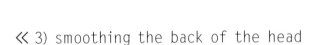

<< 3) smoothing the back of the head

Turn the head to one side, using the knot as a stabilizer. Smooth up over the back of the head and ears three times. Centralize the head, holding the knot lightly, and turn the head to the other side. Repeat the smoothing strokes three times.

4) cocooning >>

Unravel the cloth. Fold the top edge over the brow and, with a twist, down the sides of the face to the shoulders and arms, sari-fashion, to form a soft cocoon. Leave your partner to rest and assimilate the quality of your healing touches and sounds.

To finish, place a small healing crystal or flower on your partner's third eye.

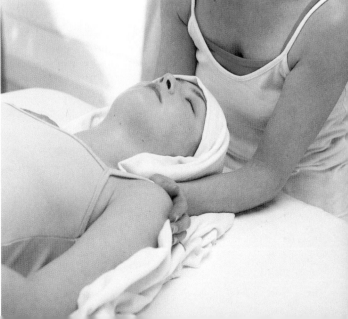

oil preparations for advanced massage

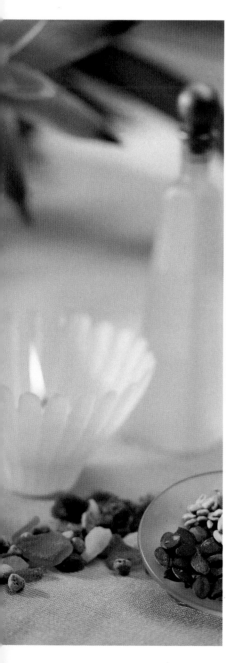

Oils are among the best nutrient sources for the skin. They contain proteins, carbohydrates and other essential ingredients which are absorbed through the openings in the hair follicles. Their effect can be quite striking since they are connected with the nerve fibres. Oil has a huge range of helpful qualities, most notably preventing dryness, increasing suppleness and delaying the effects of ageing. It softens and smoothes the skin, eliminating friction and dispersing heat evenly throughout the body.

Base or carrier oils

The best of the base or carrier oils, many of which we are familiar with as cooking mediums, are cold-pressed and virgin – a process that retains many of their trace elements and special properties. For the purposes of massage, they should be untreated by heat and free from chemical additives. I most often use the readily available and inexpensive coconut or olive oils for hair treatments – or jasmine or peach nut – and the lighter and unperfumed safflower, grapeseed, sesame and sweet almond for bodywork.

Ayurvedic preparations

Ayurvedic systems make use of some rather more exotic preparations such as mustard oil, which eases pain and swelling and wounds of all kinds; sandalwood, which helps with impotence, headaches and insomnia; bhringaraj, which prevents dandruff and dry-scalp conditions; brahmi-amla, an excellent hair-oil combination which promotes memory and helps with insomnia and sinus problems; and coriander, which removes excess body heat. These rather exotic oils are starting to make an appearance in high street bodycare stores.

The aromatherapy approach

There are numerous combinations of base oils and their more potent essential oil counterparts. Many of them can be used to treat particular afflictions of the skin, hair and body. However, the art and science of aromatherapy needs some study and should not be attempted without training. With a few rare exceptions (such as lavender and tea tree), essential oils are not used directly on the skin. Carrier or base oils must therefore be used to dilute them to safe proportions and provide the necessary lubrication to allow the masseur's hands to glide, without friction, over the skin. Essential oils can also impart their special qualities by means other than massage. I would always set the scene and create the mood for a massage either by heating or burning essential oils in a special container or, at the very least, by sprinkling them on the bedlinen or cloths I use for treatment. Their qualities are still released and affect the most primitive of our senses – smell. Sometimes, just a pierced or peeled orange can be enough.

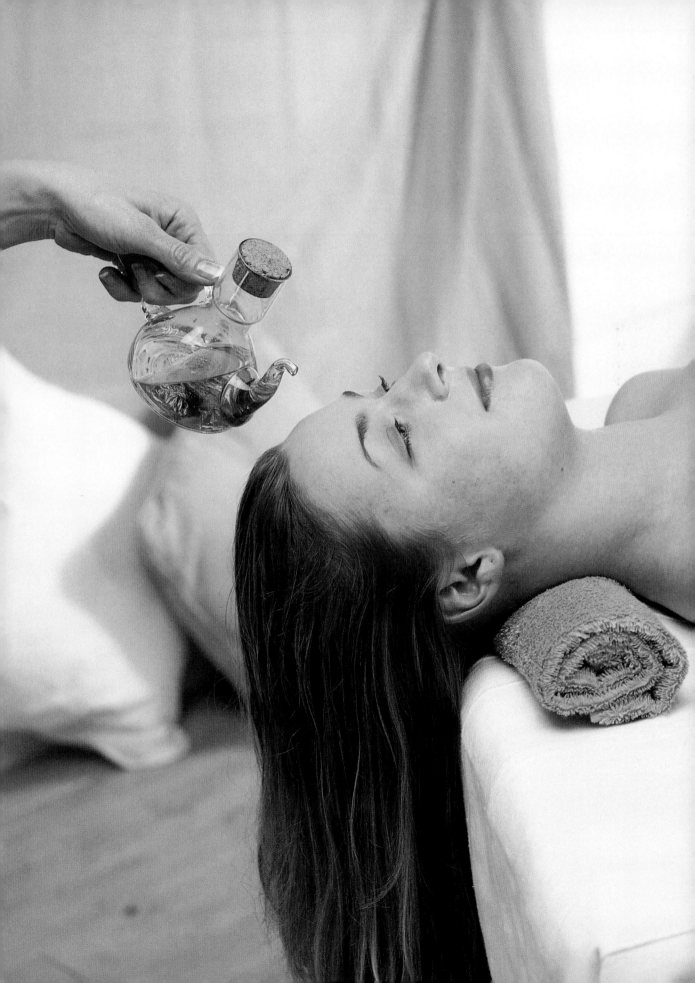

anointing the head

This is a classic treatment whose roots lie in antiquity. Use either cold-pressed virgin olive oil or your choice from a range of scented variations, warmed or at room temperature.

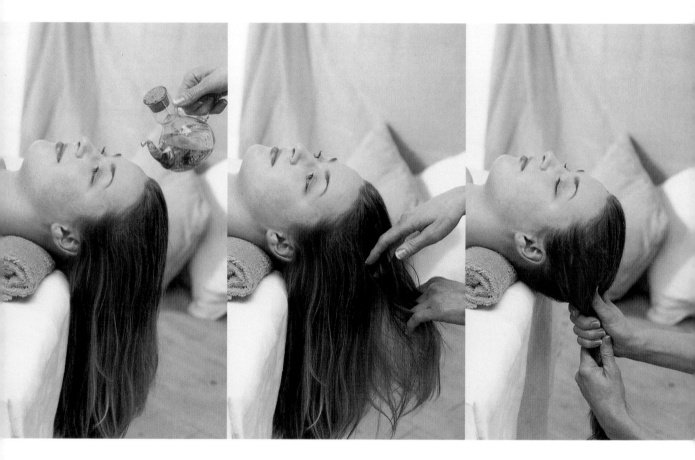

⌃ 1) Ensuring that your partner's head is well tilted back, slowly drizzle or pour the oil over the third eye and back through the hair, catching it in a bowl on the floor.

⌃ 2) Once the oil has been poured over the brow, comb through the hair with your fingers, working outwards from the scalp. Knot the hair, if long, and squeeze off the excess oil.

≫ 3) Wrap the hair in a warmed towel or make a fun foil hat by crushing tin foil around the head. Leave for several hours, if possible, to allow the oils to really penetrate into the scalp. Wash off and condition as usual.

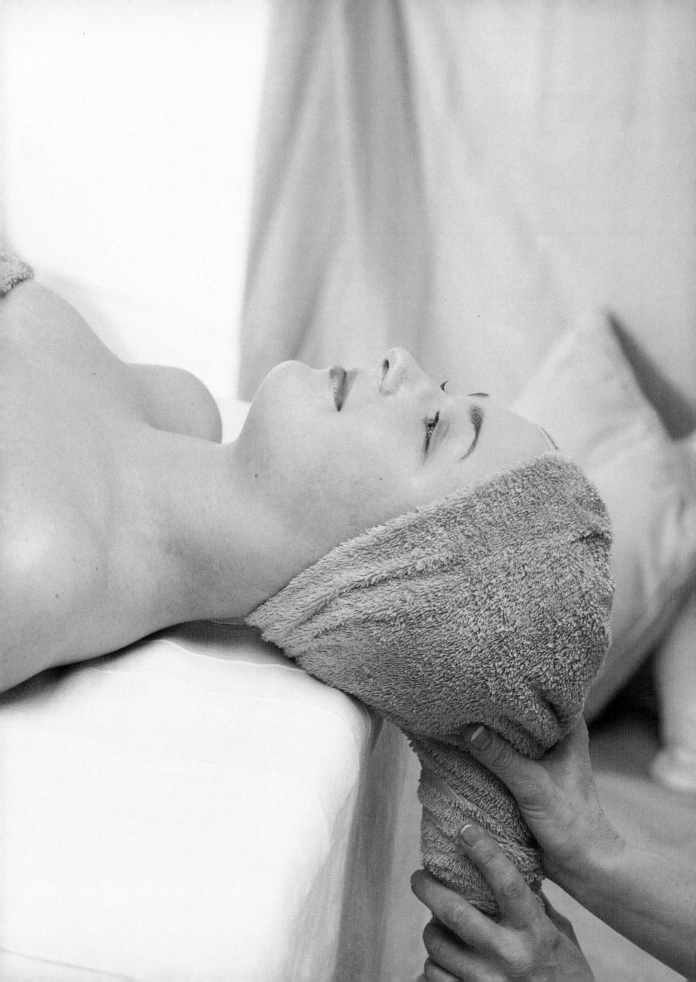

ayurvedic massage: oiling the head

Using your own choice of oil for this sequence, lubricate the three important spots – the fontanelle, the cowlick and the hollow at the base of the skull – and then spread onto the entire scalp.

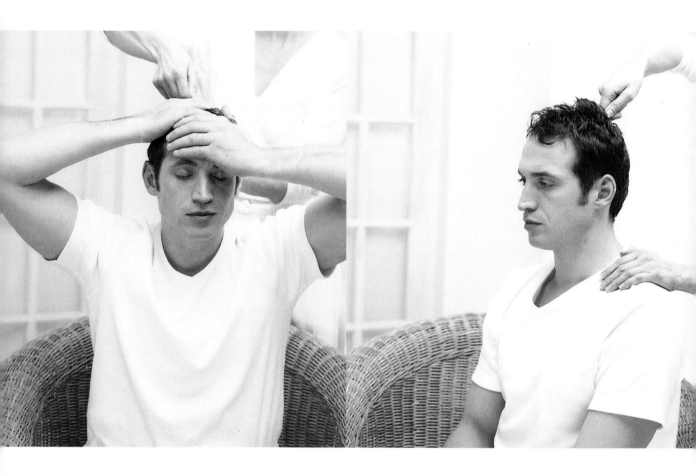

⌃1) measuring the fontanelle

Ask your partner to place their hands so that you can measure the exact location of the first point – the anterior or frontal fontanelle or *Brahmand*. With the lowest finger placed on the eyebrow centre (third eye), eight finger widths should exactly indicate the correct location of this vital point in the centre at the top of the head. One of the 10 'gates' or openings of the body, it is readily observed in babies where it is often referred to as the 'soft spot' that allows growth of the skull. When you have located this spot, rub the oil into the roots and distribute it evenly through the hair around the spot.

⌃2) locating the cowlick

Located twelve finger widths back from the eyebrow centre and physically marked by a well-defined swirl of hair, the cowlick or *Mardhi marma* is the terminating point for *Sushumna nadi* – the most important of the subtle energy channels. Traditionally this area is not shaved by Hindus and is marked by a lock of hair called a *Shikha*. As you oil this spot, twist the hair clockwise and knot it loosely together. Distribute the oil uniformly towards the temples.

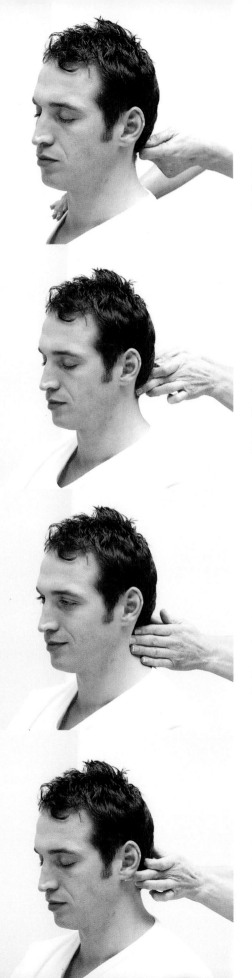

« 3) oiling the hollow

Finally, apply the oil to the third spot, the hollow at the base of the skull, where it meets the neck. Distribute the oil evenly around the area at the back of the head.

« 4) Krikatika marmas

Once all three oiling points have been addressed, locate the *Krikatika marmas* on either side of the last palpable vertebra. Massage with circular movements of the fingers.

« 5) Siramatrika marmas

Applying more oil if necessary, move on to locate the two sets of *Siramatrika marmas* on either side of the neck, just below the occiput (the bone at the back of the skull). Again massage with circular movements, removing tensions and releasing toxins.

« 6) Viduram marmas

The *Viduram marmas* are located in a depression behind the ear. Massage with circular movements continuing on the skull and around the ear until your fingers reach the temples.

Repeat steps 4, 5 and 6 in the same sequence once more.

ayurvedic massage

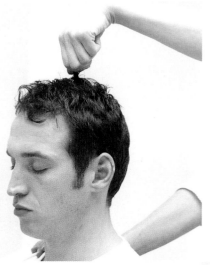

≪ 7) fontanelle: rub, twist and pull

Starting near the ears and temples, rub upwards towards the midline of the head and grasp a small amount of hair at the fontanelle or *Brahmand*. Rub, twist and pull upward with a gentle pressure in a clockwise direction. Release and repeat the action 10 times.

8) cowlick: rub, twist and pull ≫

Relocating the cowlick or *Mardhi marma*, again grasp a small amount of hair and, rubbing and twisting in a clockwise direction, pull it up with a gentle pressure. Release and repeat 10 times.

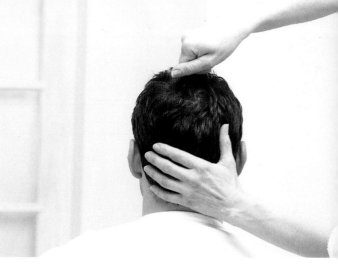

≪ 9) hollow: rub, twist and pull

Grasp a small amount of hair at the hollow at the base of the skull, and rub, twist and pull with a gentle pressure in a clockwise direction. Repeat 10 times.

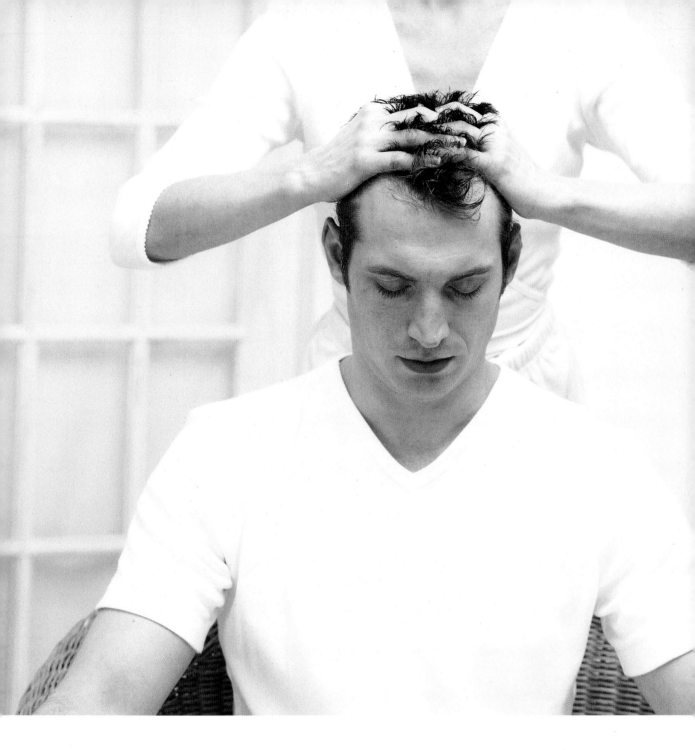

⌃ 10) complete tension release

Starting at the base of the neck, rake through the hair, smoothing through the hollow, cowlick and fontanelle and interlacing your fingers at the crown of the head. Perform the action 10 times, then shake your hands to release tension and negativities.

thai massage

In this section I have chosen to share with you some of the best techniques from the Thai and Indian traditions. They complement each other - the Thai as an introductory warm-up and the Indian as a stronger pressure method. Both help to stimulate the nerve endings. The final routine, the Tantric, reflects a non-physical approach to energy balancing.

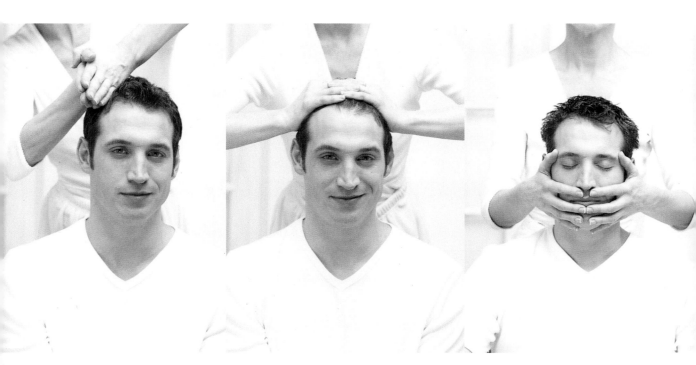

⌃1) pounding the head

Stand behind your partner and gently rest your hands on the shoulders to centre and focus your attention. Take a minute to connect to their breathing rhythms.

Place your palms together, overlapping the thumbs. Keep your wrists very relaxed as you gently 'pound' the whole of the head with the edge of your hands.

⌃2) pressing the head

Lightly interlace your fingers and 'cup' the top of the head. Gently press the heels of the hands into the sides of the head, lifting the scalp. Hold for a few seconds, release slightly and repeat two or three times.

Slide the hands around the back of the head. Press, hold and release, repeating two or three times.

Tilt the head forward and lace the hands across the back of the neck. Press, hold and release two or three times.

⌃3) cradling the face

Mould your fingers around the eyes, nose, lips and chin, holding for two or three breaths. Press gently before lightly tracing your fingers up towards the temples. Repeat two or three times.

Rest your hands back on the shoulders, allowing your partner to lean against your body for support and comfort.

4) pressing the temples »

Ensure that your partner's head is upright and support their body with yours. Place the heels of your hands in front of the ears and the palms over the temples. Slowly circle the palms away from you, six times. Circle over the cheekbones into the hollows of the cheeks to move the facial muscles.

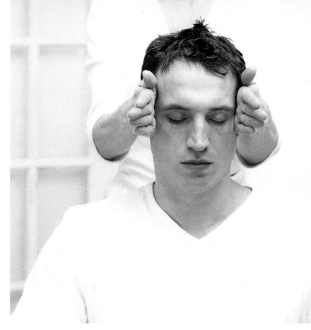

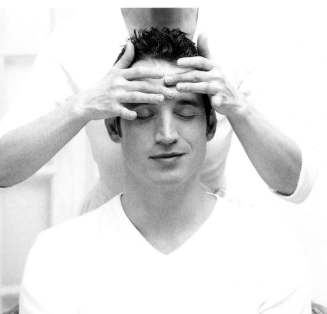

« 5) smoothing the brow

Alternating your hands, stroke your fingers upwards over the brow into the hairline, in a smoothing movement. Repeat two or three times.

6) circling and moving the scalp »

Press your fingertips into the head and, using your thumbs as levers, move the scalp in small circular movements. Lift your hands and replace your fingers on different areas of the head until you have thoroughly massaged every part.

To finish, smooth and stroke over the hair, allowing your partner to lean and rest against you for a minute.

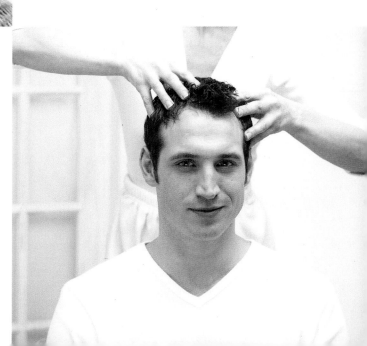

tantric healing through the chakras

As you will have gathered from the section on the subtle currents of the meridians of the Chinese and Japanese medicine systems, healing and remedial effects can be achieved without physical manipulation or massage. The Tantric system, the progenitor of all the Yoga systems of India, has its own dynamics based on a series of *chakras*, wheels of energy or lotuses, located at specific nerve plexuses along the spine. The following sequence offers a way to treat individuals who, for one reason or another, cannot easily tolerate physical massage; or it may be used as an adjunct, preparation or follow-up to other treatment forms. I have omitted interaction with *Vishuddhi* or the throat *chakra* as this could be problematical for novices.

A study of the Tantric energy systems would be very profitable for those with an interest in pursuing this ancient science. Please bear in mind that you are merely an instrument for the channelling of energy, not its source. If you have a guide or personal image of the Divine, invoke their presence for your work and do not be attached to the results. Always cleanse yourself energetically with a technique such as the waterfall (see page 31) both before and after the treatment.

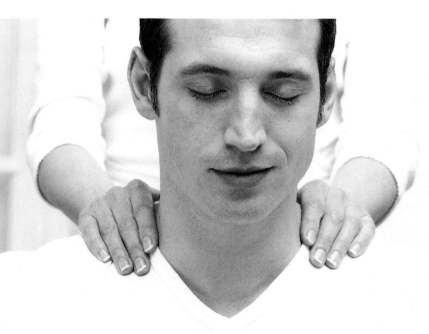

⚐ 1) making contact

As always, before starting a sequence, make sure your partner's head, neck and spine are in alignment. Since one is interacting with the most subtle and intimate aspect of another's being, I always take the precaution of asking, either explicitly or internally, for permission and guidance before starting this kind of work.

   Place your hands lightly on your partner's shoulders to make initial contact, and synchronize your breathing pattern with theirs.

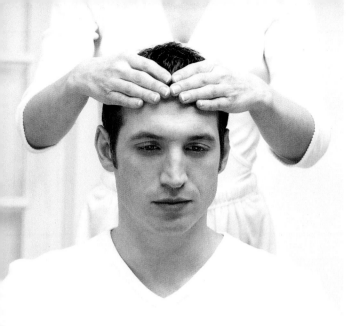

≪ 2) crowning the head: Sahasrara

The point to focus on here is located at the very crown of the head – the site of the cowlick (*mardhi marma*) and exit point of the energy channel known as *Sushumna nadi*. The gland associated with this centre is the pineal, a vestigial gland that is usually only active in children under eight years of age. I prefer not to cover the actual point itself but to encircle the area with my hands – in fact actual physical contact does not have to be made on any of these *chakras*: a hand position 2.5 cm (1 in) or so away from the head can be just as effective as you become more sensitive. As you encircle the centre, visualize a golden lotus – a perfect expression of the whole energetic being.

3) balancing Ajna chakra ≫

Ajna chakra, commonly referred to as the third eye or brow *chakra*, is the massage site of the pituitary gland, the master regulator of the endocrine system. Its proper balance ensures healthy functioning of hormones. Holding your hand in front of the centre, visualize a smokey-white two-petalled lotus, rather like an apple split in two. If you are comfortable and familiar with this *chakra's* presiding mantra or sound energy, 'Aum', silently recite it as you balance the energies.

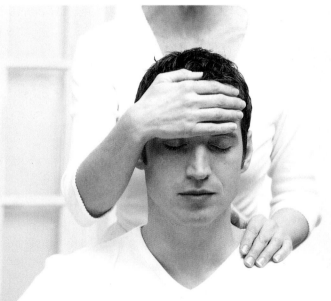

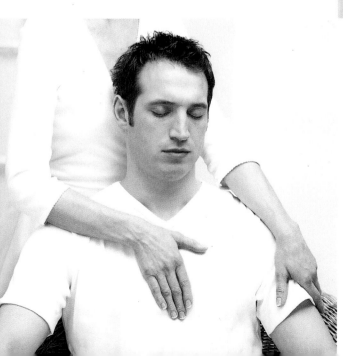

≪ 4) heart to heart: Anahata chakra

The heart centre or *Anahata chakra* is the seat of compassion and the source of the 'unstruck sound', a sound that is constant yet not made by any means. The elemental sound associated with *Anahata* is 'Yam'. Connection with this centre will make a strong energetic link with your partner and may help them to tune into the heart/compassion aspect of their being.

facial scrub and mask formulas

On that fateful day when you stare into the mirror at a lined and haggard stranger, wondering whether you could possibly justify the cost of a facelift, you may seriously have to consider some form of damage limitation. First the good news: it doesn't take plastic surgery to achieve youthful features, just a smile. This is the finest facelift of all and will not only raise your spirits but the hearts of those around you. Of course, it also helps to practise Yoga and to know how to apply some self-help massage techniques and the formulas for my scrub and mask preparations!

✱ Exfoliating facial scrub *(Suitable for all skin types)*

Ingredients 1 tsp ground almonds or fine oatmeal ✱ 1 tsp ground, dry, brown rice ✱ 3–4 tsps facial cream (if the skin is dry) or light lotion (if the skin is oily) ✱ 2–3 drops of lime or lemon juice

Method Mix the ingredients together with a small wooden spoon and apply carefully to the face with a natural bristle shaving brush. Keep your eyes closed during application and be careful not to work within the orbits of the eye sockets or directly onto the lips. As soon as the mixture has been worked into the skin and the dead cells exfoliated, rinse off very thoroughly with warm water or rosewater. Pat dry with a warmed hand towel.

✱ Fine sea salt facial scrub *(Not suitable for sensitive skin)*

Method Sprinkle 1 level tsp fine sea salt onto a warm, dampened face flannel. Keep your eyes closed and massage the salt into the face, being careful not to work into the orbits of the eye sockets or directly onto the lips. Immediately after application, rinse off very thoroughly with cold water to seal the pores. Pat dry with a hand towel.

✱ Natural astringent *(Best suited to oily skin)*

As an optional after-treatment following the fine sea-salt scrub, use crushed ripe pears as an astringent for oily skin. Using a fine cotton cloth lightly pat onto the face, be careful to avoid the orbits of the eye sockets. Leave for a few minutes for your skin to absorb the enzymes and remove any remaining excess with a cold cloth. Allow the skin to dry naturally.

✱ Fuller's Earth facial mask *(Suitable for all skin types)*

Ingredients 1 tbsp Fuller's Earth ✱ 1½–2 tbsps rosewater (for a medium to oily skin) ✱ or a small quantity of a rich face lotion (for a dry skin)

Method Make up the mask by mixing the ingredients thoroughly. Apply with a natural bristle beauty brush, avoiding the orbits of the eye sockets and the lips. If you are using rosewater, keep the mask moist with thin slices of peeled cucumber. Leave to rest for ten minutes and remove with warm rosewater. Pat dry with a fine-textured hand towel.

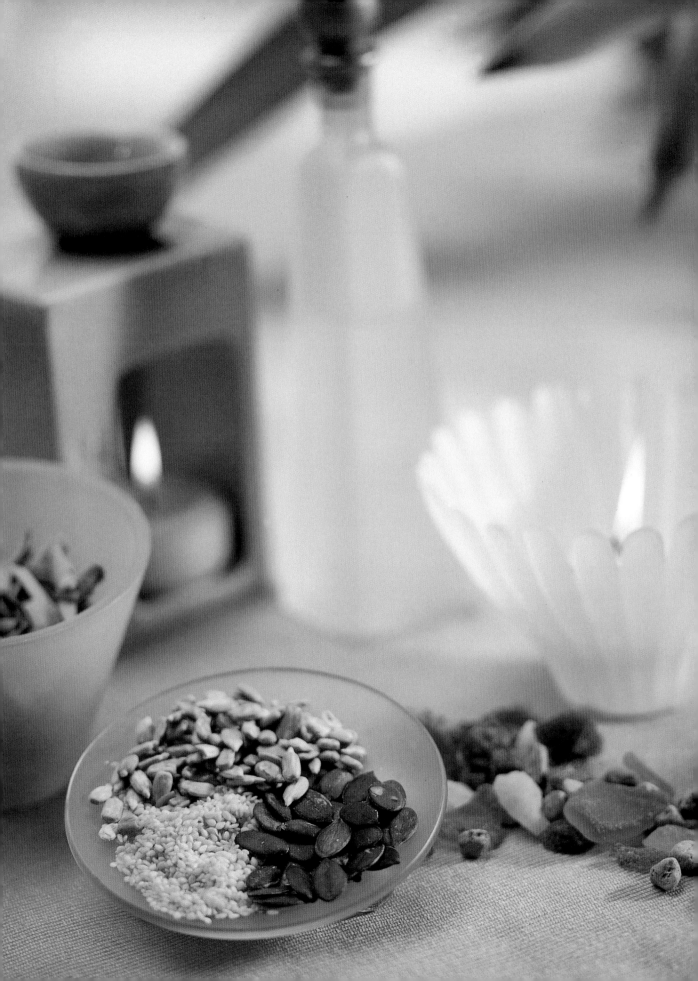

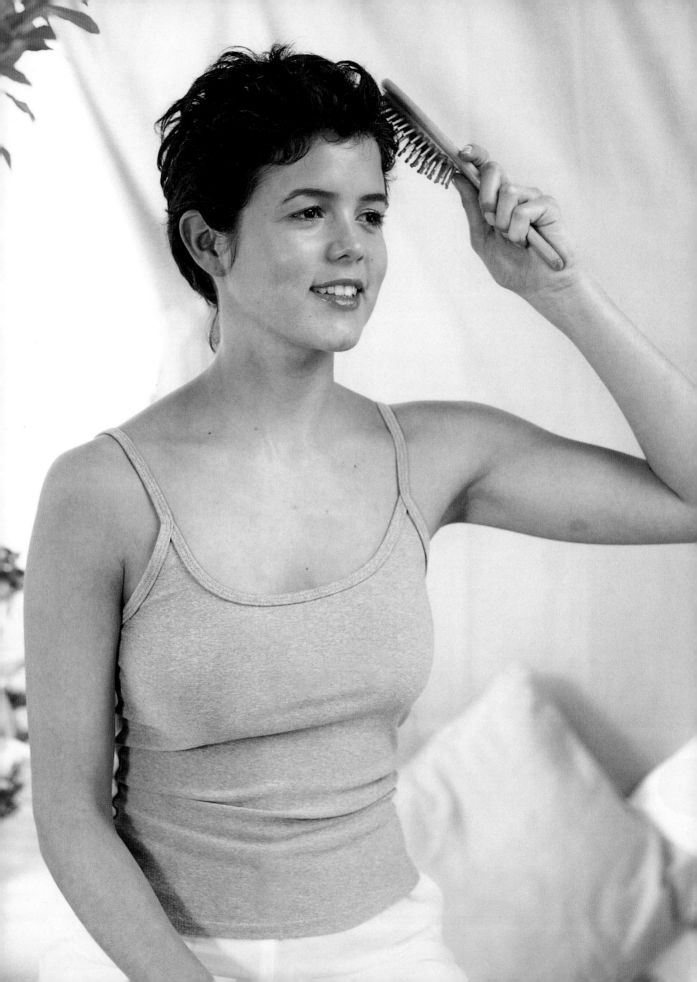

crowning glory: hair treatments

I would like to take this opportunity to indulge in a little lateral thinking. Some of the ideas outlined below might seem rather challenging, but in my experience have produced some startling results for my friends and students and are paying off in my own life.

Natural oiling

Give your hair a conditioning treatment by not washing it for several days. This will allow the natural oils to imbue the hair with a rich cocktail of self-produced minerals and sebaceous fluids. It might sound a little off-putting in a culture obsessed with frequent cleansing and shampooing, but there are ways of minimizing the sense of 'being dirty'. Pinning up longer hair is a useful cosmetic solution if you are concerned about its appearance during this trial. Brush or comb your hair twice daily and massage your scalp as often as you can to stimulate the production of your own natural bounty.

Organic products

If you colour your hair, please avoid non-organic dyes, especially peroxides. Try washing and conditioning your hair with inexpensive natural ingredients such as egg yolks (for normal to dry hair), egg whites (for oily or balanced hair), or a strong herbal infusion of camomile (for oily or balanced hair).

Washing and rinsing

Washing your hair in rainwater is very beneficial unless, of course, you live in a polluted area, in which case the rain will contain pollutants. However, if you can find a source for quality rainwater, do give this a try; you will be amazed at the results. 'Not a lot of people know this', but the final rinse after shampooing should be done with cool water - cold if you can stand it (particularly for oily hair) as it really closes the pores. Make sure you rinse thoroughly as the slightest residue of shampoo will leave the hair dull and sticky enough to attract dirt immediately.

Hot-mud treatments

There are numerous hot mud treatments on the market at the moment – a fashionable treatment that, for once, I would heartily endorse. These mineral-rich products are readily absorbed by the hair follicles and will enrich and add new lustre to tired hair.

Natural colour

For all those women of 'a certain age', why not consider letting your natural greying/silvering hair colour come through? Cast away your slavish dependence on those masking colourants. You could even perhaps take the bold step of getting your hair cut in a shorter style to remove all the damaged, discoloured and mistreated hair. A fresh start can give you so much confidence. Make a virtue of it – jump before you are pushed!

Conditioning and combing

Melted, creamed coconut or cocoa butter are hard to beat as inexpensive but very effective hair conditioners. Massage into the hair and leave for 15 minutes before shampooing and rinsing off. Another little gem: it is far better to comb your hair from the ends into the scalp in stages than draw outwards from the head which can damage the hair.

Brushing back the shine

Brush your hair thoroughly, working from the longest ends into the scalp. A routine of 50 strokes a day would be admirable. Using your fingers as a comb, dry your hair naturally without the aid of a hairdryer.

Changing your style

So many people hide behind the curtains of their hair, wondering why they have become mentally drained, depressed and physically 'stuck'. Changing one's hairstyle, even if it is brushing it in a slightly different way, can have a dramatic effect. It will change the way you feel and act and how others react to you. So, be natural and kind to your hair and it will forever be your crowning glory.

self-help hair and head massage

⌃ 1) spiralling

Using your fore- and middle fingers, rub the scalp in circular spiral movements, lifting and lightening the hair. This simple technique gives the hair 'body' and invigorates the scalp. It will recharge your batteries when your mental energies are flagging.

⌃ 2) effleurage

Using your fingertips, make small circular movements, moving the scalp away from the skull. Repeat all over the head. This often brings instant relief from tension headaches, as does simply pulling the hair close to the scalp.

⌃ 3) raking the scalp

Run your hands up over your face and rake your fingers through the hair. Repeat from the nape of the neck through to the crown of the head. This gives an instant mental relief after a concentrated day.

creating mental space

Clearing and calming your mind

Once you get on the critical path and waste time finding fault, complaining and over-explaining why you do and say certain things, the result is mental turmoil and physical exhaustion. The real downside is that people avoid your company, which creates a vicious circle, perpetuating the 'mental critic' in your head. Looking for the best outcome and the best in people is a way of starting mental space-clearing. Deciding that everything that happens is for our benefit – that we can learn from every experience – is a first step along the path of simplifying our lives. This is not an 'airy-fairy' way of seeing things because you will still be aware of the pitfalls and life consequences of actions and events – you just won't dwell on the downside of everything.

Gossiping is another habit to avoid – it is a waste of time and energy. It can become addictive in the 'waiting period' of our lives when nothing much seems to be happening. Creative interplay of ideas is far more productive and challenging. Seeing how you can help in a situation, accepting when you can't, and being detached from the outcome is a rough guide to effective time and energy management.

I have already mentioned the importance of physical space clearing and would heartily recommend Karen Kingston's books as a starting point for creating metaphysical space. This is a constant process and needs patience, persistence and quiet practice. Just get on and do what you can. It is all too easy to discover something wonderful and helpful in your life and zealously impose it on others – so watch that one, too!

A positive approach

When you have so many competing things you must do, break them down into step-by-step procedures and tackle them one by one. Be encouraged by the progress you *have* made rather than focus on all that you have *not* yet been able to achieve.

Do remember to use the positive affirmation process to repattern your way of thinking. Tantra and Yoga have always

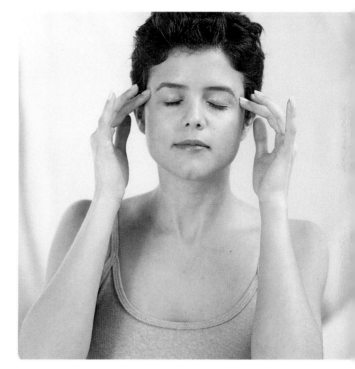

espoused the use of a short, positively worded statement – a *Sankalpa* – which addresses a short-term need or aspiration. I have plenty of evidence to show its effectiveness.

Love brings harmony and a sense of oneness with our innermost life. It is love that brings true awareness of inner peace and clears the mind so that the way ahead can be seen very clearly.

Sankalpa: thought for the day

The thought manifests as the word

The word manifests as a deed

The deed develops into habit

And the habit hardens into character

So watch the thought

And its ways with care

And let it spring from love

Born out of respect for all beings

index

acknowledgements

This book is dedicated to my mother Greta and my father Ron for gifting me the qualities, encouragement and confidence to write, and to my darling daughter, Emily, who continues to inspire my studies and teaching.

On the occasion of my first trip to Thailand, I was introduced to the shrine of the Erawan Buddha – Saan Phra Pom. Nestled in the corner of one of Bangkok's business intersections – in the lee of the luxurious Grand Hyatt Erawan Hotel – it is the focus of many Thais' affection. Local geomancers and Feng Shui experts declared this site to be sacred to Brahma, the Creator, and erected a shrine as an object of worship and veneration. This little plaza is alive from dawn to dusk with Thai folk making offerings, prayers for the health of their loved ones and lifting their hopes and loving wishes. Here, incense, flowers, and sacred dancers leave an indelible impression. It was inspiring to witness such an active spirituality and sanctuary in the everyday modern world. My partner Stephen Marriott (Tantro) and I were moved to tears by the recognition that the outer shrine is but a representation of the HeartShrine – that wellspring of loving compassion and creativity – within us all. As we offered prayers for the health of our families and friends and made positive affirmations for the achievement of our life aspirations, we fully acknowledged the forces of karmic destiny which truly shape and move the course of our lives.

I asked for continued help and support to be able to develop my life studies. This has always been forthcoming from so many kind souls to whom I lovingly offer my special thanks. In particular I wish to thank my partner and co-writer Stephen Marriott for his continued loving and creative support; my daughter Emily, who was such a beautiful and hard-working model on all the photo-shoots and continues to be my supportive soulmate; my close friend and confidant Sam Southall, photographer, for all his wonderful developmental work and the most fun, productive and creative photo-shoots in town; Bonny Andrews and Colin Day and their charming daughters, Jo and Clo – the junior models in this book – for their unstinting support and professional attitude; Charles and Lara Tibbetts for all their help and modelling skills; Zoe Daino for her willingness to allow her beauty to shine as a model and for great set design; Anna Blain for her friendship and for sharing her skills as a masseur; Sue Gowen who kindly modelled during her massage treatment; Pam Griffith for her stunning art backgrounds; Sue and Malcolm Wilcox for so generously granting access to their beautiful home for our first pre-shoot; Donald Henderson for the use of Stourbridge Coach House during the second pre-shoot; Claire Harvey and Robert Hewett for their patient modelling at the final photo-shoot; Karen O'Grady for her supportive role; my dear friends Eileen Paradise and Ann Jennings for loans of props; photographer Jacqui Wornell for the final photo-shoot; Donna Allen for her spirit, brilliant make-up, hair styling and the entrée to Mo-Mo's restaurant; Wax Lyrical for the kind loan of ceramics, candles and bases; and especially Mark Duff's 'new-concept treatment couches' for the wonderful on-site massage chair and valuable remedial accessories used in the book – a must for any professional practitioner (tel: 01473 720572, email: www. new concept. co.uk). Many thanks also go to Jane McIntosh at Hamlyn for her steadfast support through the creation of the book. Thanks to Random House publisher for permission to use elements of Joseph Corvo's *Zone Therapy* book. Finally I acknowledge and thank the many friends and students who have taught me so much over the years and are the real reason for the work I do.